I0125602

healthy feet

FOR PEOPLE WITH DIABETES

DR. MARK HINKES, DPM

Doctor of Podiatric Medicine

dr-mark.net

Healthy Feet for People With Diabetes

Copyright ©2012 by Mark Hinkes, DPM

Page Design and Production by Picante Creative

Cover Design by Gisela Swift

Edited by Judy Stanton

Medical Photos by Mark Hinkes, DPM

All rights reserved. Printed in the United States of America.
No part of this book may be reproduced or transmitted in any
form or by any means, electronic or mechanical including photocopying,
recording, or by information storage and retrieval system without
written permission from the publisher except for the inclusion
of brief quotations in articles and reviews.

This information is not intended to replace the attention or advice
of a physician or other healthcare professional.

....

Library of Congress cataloging-in-publication data
Hinkes, Dr. Mark,
Healthy Feet for People With Diabetes/ Dr. Mark Hinkes
ISBN-13: 978-0-9856286-0-4
ISBN-10: 098562860X
Medical
Web Site: www.dr-mark.net
Copyright Registered: 2012
First Published by HealthyFeet, LLC in the USA
June 2012

DEDICATION

To my patients, whom I have had
the privilege to serve and learn from.

In Memory of Laura Jacobs, MD, PhD. My mentor,
my teacher, a person who loved people and dedicated
herself to making their lives better. Her work has
left the world a better place than she found it.

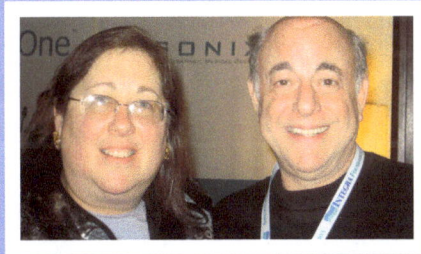

ENDORSEMENTS

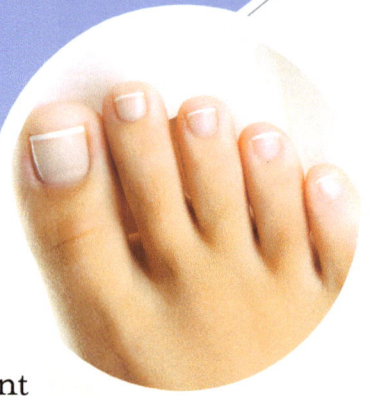

Healthy Feet for People With Diabetes is an excellent book on diabetic foot care. In my opinion, these 100+ pages should be read by all —be he or she a doctor, nurse, caregiver or sufferer; there is a lot for everyone to learn from this book. The book nicely covers various aspects of foot care. There are elaborate chapters on nail care, skin care, basic foot hygiene, shoes and socks. Information from these chapters will help prevent diabetic foot lesions. Chapters on infection, ulcers and common foot problems educate one regarding management of foot conditions. The chapter on the medical team gives one a clear idea regarding the people involved from different specialties in rendering foot care. It will definitely enlighten many and will go a long way in contributing to diabetic foot amputation prevention. Hardly ever have I found any author writing about medical issues simply enough to keep the text understandable by all readers. This aspect has especially fascinated me. I congratulate Mark for compiling such a beautiful piece of literature.

— Dr. Kshitij Shankhdhar MD, Dip.Diab., FAPWCA, FICN, Diabetologist and Diabetic Foot Expert, L.K.Diabetes Centre, Lucknow, India.

"Wow! Dr. Hinkes does it again! He makes understanding Diabetes and Diabetic Feet so SIMPLE. Every issue and question is uncovered in this thoughtful, comprehensive and insightful book. It should be on the book shelf of every diabetic patient as well as every clinician who treats these individuals!"

— Cynthia Ann Fleck, RN, BSN, MBA, ET/WOCN, APN/CNS, CWS, CFCN, DNC, St. Louis, MO.

At the time of my first visit to Dr. Hinkes, my feet had numerous sores, due to the fact that I was overweight and suffered from unmanaged diabetes. The doctor examined my feet and told me that while he was the physician, it was up to me — and nobody else — to turn my eating habits around and get my diabetes under control. I took him at his word, went on a low-carb diet and started checking my blood sugar three times a day. As a result, my feet are doing much better, I've lost 55 pounds, my blood sugar levels have improved, and I feel healthier overall.

Had it not been for Dr. Hinkes, I never would have made those important changes to improve my health, and I'm very fortunate to have access to his medical expertise.

— Bill Cole, Nashville, TN.

Healthy Feet for People With Diabetes is the follow up book to Dr. Hinkes' first book, *Keep The Legs You Stand On*. *Healthy Feet* is a considerably shorter book than his first work, but it is packed with information on foot health that is vital for people with diabetes. Dr. Hinkes has taken a rather dry and mundane subject and given it life to benefit people with diabetes by encouraging them to learn about foot health to prevent triggering events that can lead to foot ulcers, infections, and amputations. The design of the book makes it easy-to-read, even for people who may be visually impaired, and holds the reader's interest from first page to last. The resources section of the book provides additional sources of valuable information and resources for general and foot health. In this time of growing numbers of people with diabetes and at risk limbs, education on prevention leading to healthy feet is the logical way approach a problem that is fast becoming epidemic in proportion and offers a cost-effective solution. This book is a must-read for patients with diabetes and their caregivers who wish to learn how to care for their feet and prevent the complications of diabetes to their feet.

— The late Laura Jacobs, MD, PhD., Newton Centre, MA.

Amputation of the legs is one of the most common complications of diabetes — yet is still one frequently ignored by health care providers. In most cases, diabetics are counseled on the potential dangers of renal failure, premature heart disease and retinopathy, among others, but rarely are foot care and foot complications included as part of this education.

Written in a very friendly caregiver-to-patient format, Dr. Hinkes directly addresses the main concerns of diabetics related to foot care, using recommendations fully backed by scientific evidence.

The book is very thorough and complete, starting with fundamental topics including hygiene, exercise, shoes and socks, but also provides a wealth of information on other topics, such as how to recognize foot problems and complications early.

I am convinced that all those with diabetes should read this book to help achieve Dr. Hinkes' goal of keeping diabetics' feet healthy. Without question, the book is a must-have reference for both health care providers and diabetes patients all around the world.

— Jose Contreras-Ruiz, M.D., Director, Interdisciplinary Wound and Ostomy Care Center, Dr. Manuel Gea Gonzalez General Hospital, Mexico City, Mexico.

Healthy Feet for People with Diabetes is an excellent resource for those who want to be more proactive in foot health, especially when faced with the diagnosis of diabetes or pre-diabetes. This follow-up to Dr. Hinkes' first book *Keep the Legs You Stand On* is a must-read as well as an essential resource for patients, families, medical students and practitioners alike who comprise the multidisciplinary team involved in the many aspects of intervention and treatment of individuals with diabetes. As a podiatric physician, I have seen firsthand what 'not knowing' can do to those who suffer from peripheral diabetic neuropathy and I commend and applaud Dr. Hinkes as he succinctly and clearly explains the "do's and don'ts" to follow for proper foot health. Individuals with diabetes as well as their family members will feel empowered with the information that Dr. Hinkes shares with them. I would encourage both local as well as national organizations like the American Diabetes Association and Juvenile Diabetes Research Foundation to adopt this handbook and offer it as a resource tool available to a recent or long-standing diagnosed individual of Type 1 or Type 2 diabetes. With regards to greater emphasis being placed on prevention of chronic disease in our health care arena today, Dr. Hinkes successfully presents us with the gift of knowledge and practical tips and tools easily applied to everyday life. In the words of Atul Gawande, MD, *"Betterment is a perpetual labor...."* and the driving force behind Dr. Hinkes' commitment and labor of love is to better the lives of those afflicted with diabetes by empowering them with simple steps towards foot health and amputation prevention. Kudos, Dr. Hinkes!

— Kathya M. Zinszer, D.P.M., F.A.P.W.C.A., Temple University, Philadelphia, Pennsylvania.

If I would have taken the time to seek Podiatric care instead of doing my own (diabetic) foot care (I had knowledge about foot care, but not enough), I might not have lost my leg. I was hardheaded and proud, so I did not go to the doctor because I thought I could take care of my foot problem myself.

Dr. Hinkes educated me on how important it is to take care of my feet because of my diabetes. I know now what I should have known then about my feet. I will encourage any person with diabetes to seek professional help when it comes to their feet.

— Michael Hinton, Clarksville, TN.

Healthy Feet for People with Diabetes is THE comprehensive guide and users manual on what to do and what not to do with, for, and to the feet, for people with diabetes. It clearly and easily explains the "why's" and "why nots," and makes easy sense of this otherwise complicated issue.

A must-read for anyone with diabetes, and a highly recommended reference for those on the patient health care team.

We only get one pair of feet and we have to keep them healthy in order to carry us through our life's journeys. As a follow-up to *Keep the Legs You Stand On*, Dr. Hinkes has once again done his best to educate all of us on proper foot care so that all our travels are "problem free"!

— Howard Green, DPM, D.A.B.P.S., F.A.C.F.A.S., Head, Dept of Podiatry & Immediate Past-Director of Post-Graduate, Podiatric Surgical Residency Training Vancouver General Hospital / University of British Columbia, Private Practice, Surrey, BC, www.drhowardgreen.com

DISCLAIMER

This book is a guide to assist people with diabetes and their caregivers with clinical and educational information on prevention of foot ulcers, infections and amputations. It is designed for informational purposes only and is not intended to substitute for professional medical advice, diagnosis, or treatment. People with diabetes should never disregard professional medical advice because of information in this book. The author is not responsible or liable for any damage or loss resulting from medical evaluations, recommendations, or medical treatments listed here. Always consult with your medical professional for individual patient evaluation, treatment, or recommendations. Reliance on this information without consultation with a qualified medical professional is at your own risk.

In a medical emergency, call your doctor or 911 immediately.

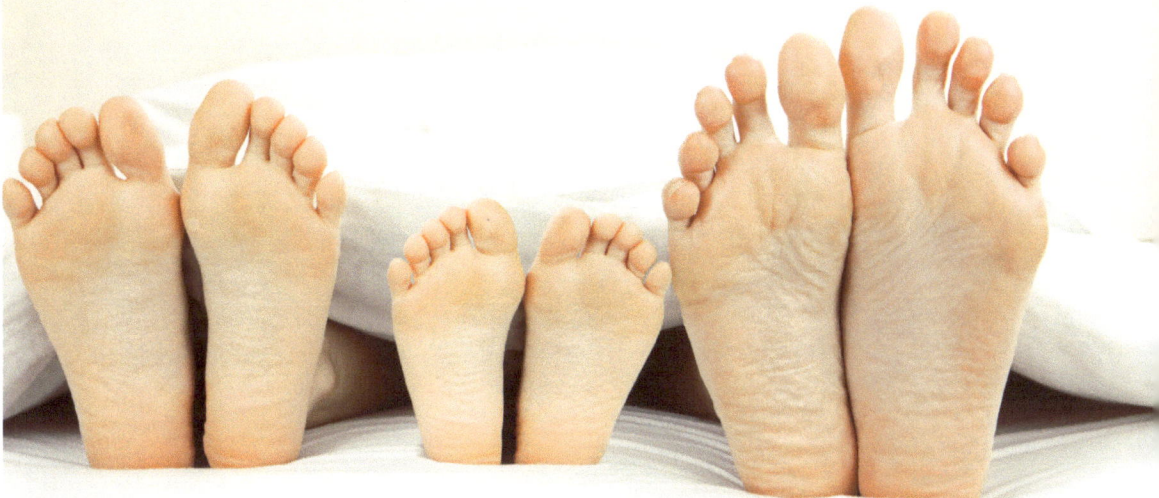

TABLE OF CONTENTS

TABLE OF CONTENTS

A highly-prized seafood delicacy found in the Gulf of Mexico in South Florida is the stone crab. The only portion of the crab that is harvested is the claw, as it contains a delicious sweet white meat. Only one claw is harvested at a time. With its one remaining claw, the stone crab can still defend itself from predators while it re-grows the missing claw. Unfortunately, this is not the case with your feet. Your feet are not replaceable. As the American Podiatric Medical Association says, "Feet must last a lifetime."

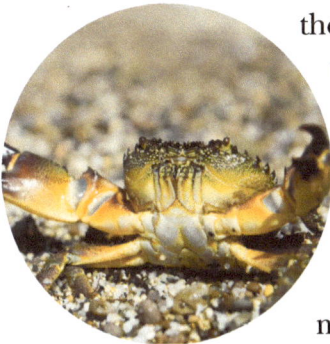

As a foot doctor for people with diabetes, every day of my working life is spent seeing people perhaps like you suffer with the complications of diabetes to their feet. This book was borne out of my frustration at observing people needlessly endure debilitating foot ulcers, infections and even amputations because they lack education and fail to practice preventive behaviors that result in healthy feet.

Unfortunately, most people don't go to the doctor until they are in pain or fear for their health. The medical profession has made some progress in making the public aware of the importance of going to the doctor for the purpose of prevention — such as in getting routine pap smears, mammograms, prostate exams, eye exams, dental check-ups and teeth cleanings, treadmill stress tests, colonoscopies and physical exams.

Since you are reading this book, you have already taken the first step towards addressing your foot health before it gets out of control. As a person with diabetes, it is essential that you *add a yearly foot exam with a monofilament test to your list of preventive health screenings.*

Through this book, I hope you will learn how diabetes can affect your feet and legs and that you will gain insight into how to prevent and overcome your foot health problems by practicing preventive foot health behaviors. The care of your feet is in your hands; with this information, it is up to you to create your personal prevention strategy to promote good foot health.

It isn't easy for a doctor to consistently use lay terminology to describe complex medical conditions, but I have made every effort to explain the issues of the diabetic foot and foot care in the simplest possible terms.

There are many good resources online and in print to provide you with additional information and medical terms. Most importantly, ASK YOUR DOCTOR when you don't understand something; educating you is an important part of his or her job.

Still, YOU are the most important person on your health care team. While your doctors, nurses and therapists can give you advice and direction, it is up to you to take the necessary actions to increase your chances of living a healthy, normal life.

Mark Hinkes, DPM

George Bernard Shaw wrote, "I marvel that society would pay a surgeon such a large sum of money to remove a person's leg, but nothing to save it." Because of the mixed incentives, prevention of amputations is not often given valid consideration. *Healthy Feet for People with Diabetes* arms patients with vital information to prevent their own amputation.

We know the statistics are staggering. Diabetes affects 26 million Americans and an additional 79 million more have a condition called pre-diabetes — that's one-third of the population. Up to 25% of those with diabetes will get a foot ulcer. A foot ulcer is the most common reason for a diabetic admission to the hospital and the most common factor leading to an amputation. Every 30 seconds, somewhere in the world a limb is lost as a consequence of diabetes.

But it doesn't have to end that way. We know what causes ulcers and amputations. We have interventions to prevent that natural progression. Unfortunately, the specialty of limb salvage or amputation prevention is in its infancy, so patients have to be proactive in seeking qualified care.

In *Keep the Legs You Stand On*, Dr. Mark Hinkes provided an owners manual to the diabetic foot. In this book, he expands upon that manual and with conciseness he explains the most important steps people with diabetes can take towards preventing foot complications and potential amputations. Diabetes doesn't have to mean you have one foot in the grave.

Lee C. Rogers, D.P.M.
Director, Amputation Prevention Center, Van Nuys, CA
Past Chair, Foot Care Council, American Diabetes Association

CHAPTER 1

DIABETES AND YOUR FEET

A journey of one thousand
miles begins with the first step.

— **Lao-tzu,** *The Way of Lao-tzu*
Chinese philosopher (604 BC –531 BC)

When you were diagnosed with diabetes, your doctor and other health care providers probably talked with you about this health condition and gave you educational materials to help you better understand the impact this disease has on your body.

This book focuses specifically on the foot problems faced by people with diabetes. Like all complications of diabetes, foot problems are better controlled when your blood sugar is controlled.

Chronically elevated blood sugars cause damage to your nerves and blood vessels. The smallest arteries, called arterioles, that circulate blood to your extremities and organs, become narrowed or blocked.

When this happens, the nerves that the arteries serve are deprived of the fresh oxygenated blood and nutrients needed to function normally. Over time, the nerves will fail.

The results of nerve failure include loss of vision, loss of kidney function, and loss of protective sensation for pain in the foot, also known as "diabetic sensory neuropathy." This condition leaves your foot vulnerable to painless or silent trauma that can lead to foot ulcers, infections, hospitalizations and amputations.

So, if you do a good job of controlling your blood sugars, you will be less likely to develop foot problems.

The foot is a very sturdy structure. You need healthy feet to remain active and independent. While everyone's feet are subject to physical forces, stresses, and deformities, people with diabetes must be even more vigilant about foot care. As a person with diabetes, your body responds different-

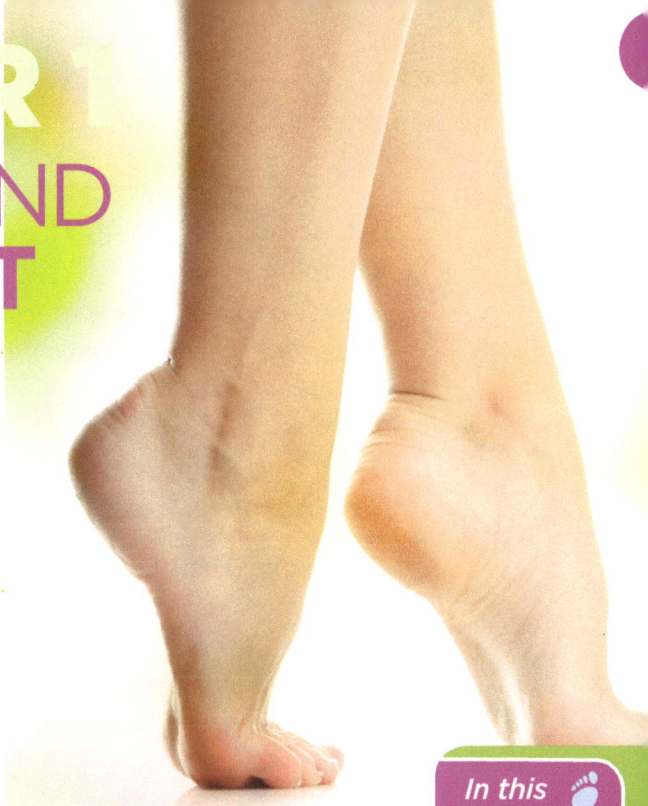

In this chapter

WARNING
SIGNS
OF FOOT
PROBLEMS

DIABETIC
FOOT RISK
CLASSIF-
ICATION
SYSTEM

ly than the average person, and you are at higher risk to develop complications.

Please, don't take your feet for granted. It's better to know than to be sorry.

TOP TIPS Warning Signs Of Foot Problems

✓

WARNING SIGNS OF FOOT PROBLEMS

Swelling

Temperature

Color changes

Pain

LOPS

Cramps

Numbness

Wounds

In-grown Toenails

Corns and Calluses

Hair

Bony Bumps

Shape Change

Balance

Rash

Dry Skin

If you experience any of the following symptoms, this is your body giving you a *warning sign that your foot is at risk and you need to seek professional foot care*. Common foot problems that might normally seem to be a minor disturbance can quickly turn into a major health issue for people with diabetes.

- **Swelling:** foot or ankle swelling

- **Temperature:** cold feet or legs; increased warmth

- **Color changes:** redness, skin color changes or discolored, streaked or thickened toenails

- **Pain:** leg pain, especially when wearing shoes; pain on the inside of your arch or the bottom of your heel; soreness when you step out of bed in the morning; any persistent pain; burning feeling in your feet; even pain when at rest or while walking

- **LOPS:** loss of protective sensation for pain; that is, the

loss of the ability to feel pain in your feet

- **Cramps:** cramps in your leg when you walk; painful cramps in the toes

- **Numbness:** numbness in your feet

- **Open Sores:** even small ones, with or without drainage

- **Wounds:** especially those on your foot or leg that do not heal promptly

- **In-grown toenails:** sides of toenails digging into skin that may hurt

- **Calluses and corns:** whether painful or painless, calluses on the bottom of the foot or corns on the toes

- **Hair:** lack of hair growing on foot

- **Bony Bumps:** bones that stick out, such as large bony bumps behind the big toe on the inside of the foot, or large bony bumps behind the small toe on the outside of the foot

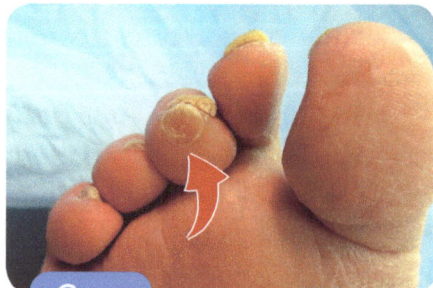
Corn

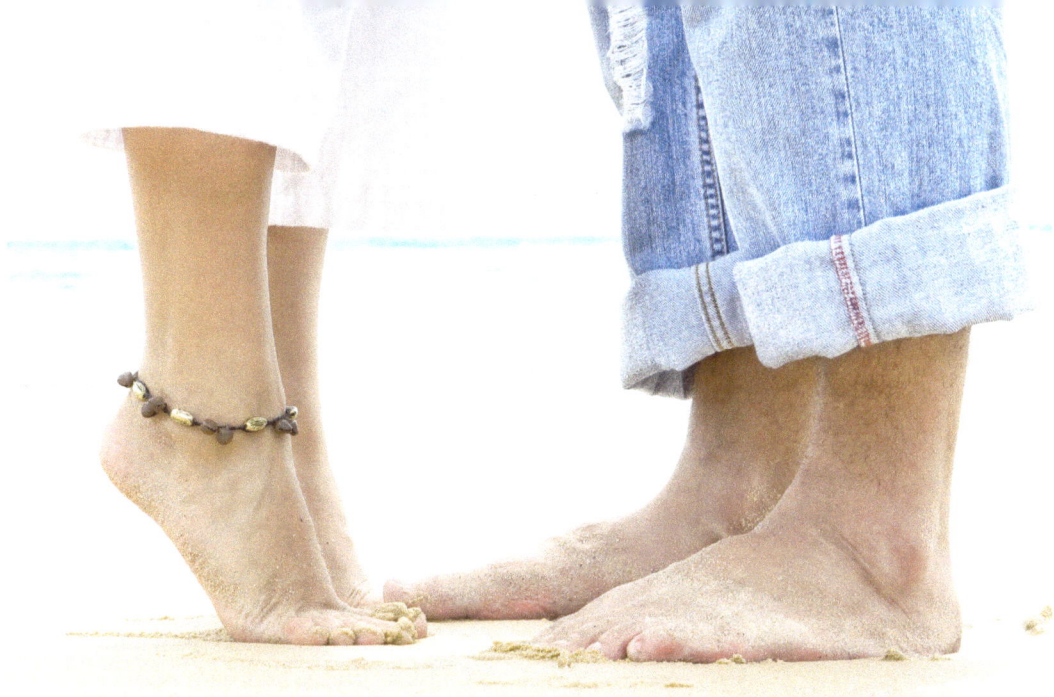

- **Shape changes:** change in the size or shape of your foot or ankle, toes that are cocked up or bent, or a deformity of the mid-foot

- **Balance:** loss of balance or falling because you cannot feel the floor with your feet

- **Rash:** skin rash

- **Dry, scaly skin:** feet that are always dry and scaly and sometimes itch

DIABETIC FOOT RISK CLASSIFICATION SYSTEM:
Where Do You Stand?

To keep the legs you stand on, it might help for you to better understand your "risk" for having a foot ulcer or worse, an amputation. 85% of all lower extremity amputations start with a foot ulcer. So, preventing the ulcer almost guarantees keep-

85% OF ALL LOWER EXTREMITY AMPUTATIONS START WITH A FOOT ULCER.

ing your foot and leg. When you look at this classification system, think about yourself and where you fit. Then, read the recommendations for "ongoing care." If you follow those recommendations, you can reduce your risk. These guidelines were developed by The International Working Group on the Diabetic Foot (IWGDF) and are accepted worldwide.

To understand your risk for developing a foot ulcer, you must first have a foot exam to determine whether or not you have protective sensation for pain with your feet. This is normally done with a monofilament-testing device. If you do not feel the monofilament testing device, you have what is called Loss of Protective Sensation for Pain (LOPS). The number listed next to the Risk Category represents your "odds" of developing a foot ulcer. LOPS can be a "trigger" towards developing a foot ulcer and ultimately needing an amputation.

Risk Category 0
Foot Ulcer Risk Odds = 0/1

SYMPTOMS:

This is the lowest-risk for a person with diabetes. You are in this category if you CAN feel the monofilament-testing device and have what is called "protective sensation for pain." You have no history of a foot ulcer and no foot deformity.

ONGOING CARE:

You should be educated about diabetes, practice preventive foot care behaviors, keep your blood sugars under control and see a foot care specialist once a year for reevaluation.

If you DO NOT have the ability to sense pain in your foot, you have what is called LOPS or "loss of protective sensation for pain." That places you in one of the three following categories. A foot health history by a foot care specialist and foot examination will help define your specific foot

problems of the bones, soft tissues, and nails and place you in the correct category.

Risk Category 1
Foot Ulcer Risk Odds = 1.7/1

SYMPTOMS:

You are in this category if you have lost protective sensation for pain, but have no foot deformities or history of ulcers to your feet.

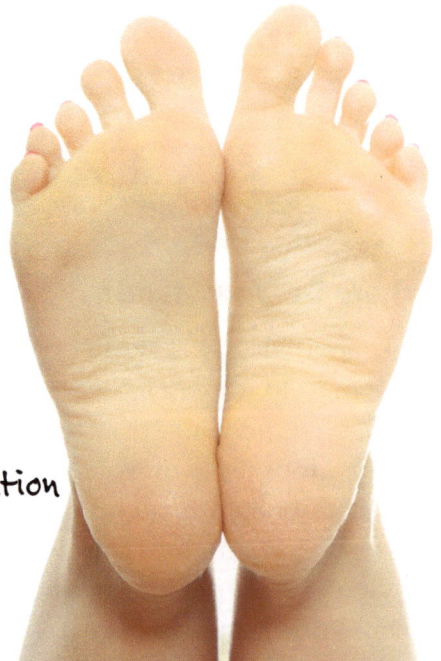

ONGOING CARE:

You should be educated about diabetes, practice preventive foot care behaviors, control your blood sugars, and see a foot care specialist once a year for reevaluation. You will be encouraged NOT to walk barefooted, and may be advised to wear a preven-

☑

LOPS

Loss Of Protective Sensation For Pain

category 1 - have lost protective sensation for pain, but have no foot deformities or history of ulcers to your feet.

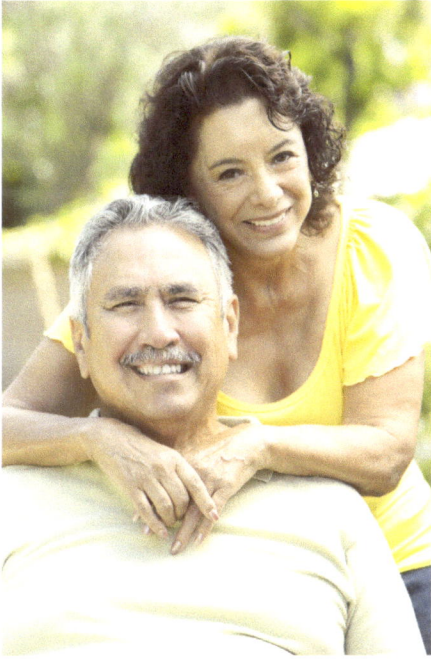

ACCORDING TO THE AMERICAN DIABETES ASSOCIATION, DIABETES AFFECTS **27 MILLION PEOPLE IN THE US** AND 330 MILLION PEOPLE WORLDWIDE.

FACTS

tive, cushioned insole for shock absorption and protection from shearing forces against the foot.

Risk Category 2
Foot Ulcer Risk Odds = 12.1/1

SYMPTOMS:

You are in this category if you have lost protective sensation for pain and have a foot deformity of the bones, soft tissues, or nails.

ONGOING CARE:

You should be educated about diabetes, practice preventive foot behaviors, control your blood sugars, and see a foot care specialist several times a year. You may benefit from insoles or custom-made biomechanical orthotics and/or special diabetic

shoes to relieve pressure or to accommodate a deformed foot. For your callus, corn, and nail trimming, you should use the services of a foot care specialist, especially if you also have poor vision or hand-eye coordination.

Risk Category 3
Foot Ulcer Risk Odds = 36.4/1

SYMPTOMS:

If you are in this category, you are at the highest risk for foot ulcers, infections and amputation. You have lost protective sensation for pain and you may have a history of a previous foot ulcer, bone infection, amputation, Charcot Foot, circulation problems, gangrene, or a diagnosis of kidney disease.

ONGOING CARE:

You should be seen by a foot care specialist at least every two months, depending on your needs. You will be evaluated for insoles, shoes, braces, or the appropriate treatment for your foot health needs and ongoing foot care.

On this website, (www.dr-mark.net), you can find more information that can help you to identify your risk factors for foot ulcers, infections, and amputations and provide recommendations for prevention and educational information to help you maintain good foot health.

Monofilament Testing

INSTRUCTIONS

(If you can't see the bottom of your feet, use a mirror or ask someone to help you.)

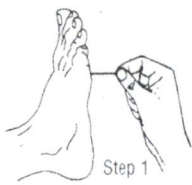

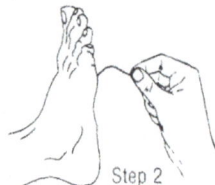

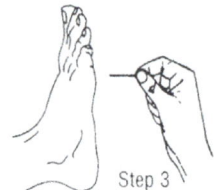

Step 1   Step 2   Step 3

1. Hold the red filament by the paper handle (see step 1 picture above).

2. Touch the filament to the skin at each site for only 1-2 seconds. Touch near the side of, and NOT directly on, an ulcer, a callous, or scar. Push to make the filament bend (see step 2 picture above).

If you do not feel the monofilament when you touch your foot, you have LOPS.

CHAPTER 2
HEALTHY FOOT HABITS

An ounce of prevention is worth a pound of cure.

— Benjamin Franklin

① Prevention

The American Diabetes Association (ADA) recommends that annual foot risk screenings begin five years after you are diagnosed with diabetes. However, it is never too early to develop good foot health habits. By taking care of your feet every day, you can often prevent diabetic foot complications. While it is important to take care of your overall health, it is just as important to seek care for your feet as soon as you suspect you might need it.

So, if you read nothing else in this book, read this. It's a good overview of preventive footcare behaviors and what you should do to keep your feet healthy. The following chapters go into further details on these key elements of foot care.

TOP TIPS

① DAILY INSPECTION: Look at and touch your feet every day: from top to bottom, the back, the side, and even between the toes. You are inspecting your feet for cuts, blisters, redness, and a local increase in temperature, swelling or nail problems. If you run your hands over your feet daily, you will learn the feel of your foot and will be able to pick up changes.

If you have difficulty seeing your feet, pick good lighting, wear glasses or try using a magnifying hand mirror to see the bottom of your feet. You can put your foot up on your knee or rest it on a foot stool where it can be closer to your eyes. If nothing else works, ask another person to look at your feet.

If you find corns, calluses, redness, pus, swelling, sores, or cracks in the skin; if you have

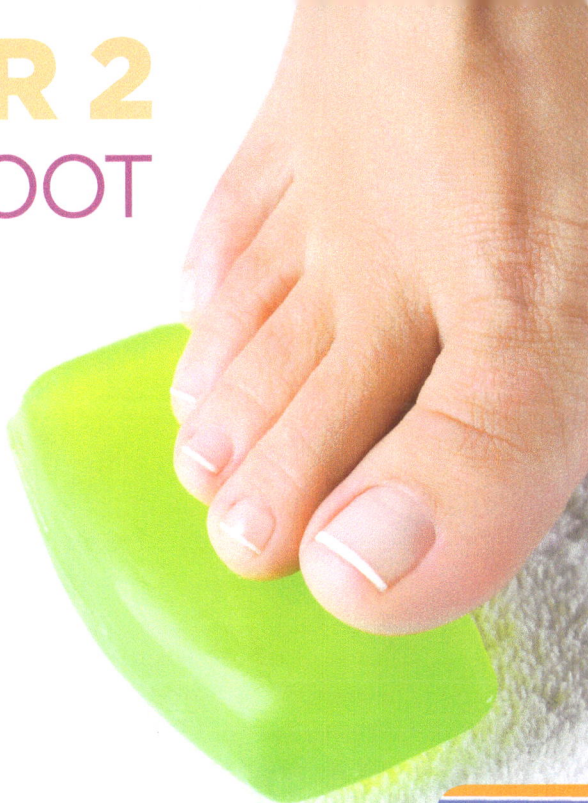

In this chapter

PREVENTION

BASIC FOOT
HYGIENE:
WASHING
YOUR FEET

pain; or if you see anything unusual, immediately consult your doctor or foot care specialist and get prompt medical attention for any problems.

2 DAILY WASHING. Gently wash your feet with soap in lukewarm (not hot) water — the temperature you would use on a newborn baby — using a soft cloth or sponge. Pay special attention to the space between the toes. Do not soak sore feet. Get professional attention to identify small problems before they turn into big problems.

3 DRYING FEET. Always keep your feet clean and dry. After you wash them, dry your feet carefully and thoroughly, especially between the toes, before you put on your socks and shoes. Never rub the feet vigorously. If your feet tend to sweat, apply a mild foot powder or baby powder after washing and drying carefully. Prescription medications are available for nonresponsive cases of foot perspiration.

4 MOISTURIZING. If your skin is dry, moisturize it daily to prevent itching or cracking. Do not use moisturizer between the toes or around the toenails; this could encourage infection. Wait until your skin is dry to apply moisturizer. Soften your skin by massaging your feet with a lanolin or urea-based lotion or cream.

5 NAIL CARE. Cut your nails carefully, and then file the sharp edges to smooth them. Follow the shape of the toe, cutting straight across without clipping the corners, which could cause the nail to become ingrown. It's best to trim nails when they are soft after bathing and to use a good light. If your nails are too thick or tend to split or crack when trimming, have your podiatrist cut them for you.

6 TREATING COMMON FOOT PROBLEMS. To avoid injury to your feet, do not trim corns, calluses or ingrown toenails; or pick at loose skin, warts, corns, or calluses; or pop open any blisters.

Have them treated by your doctor or a foot care professional. Do not use over-the-counter medicines such as ingrown toenail remover; corn, callus, or wart remover; or medicated foot pads that contain salicylic acid. These treatments are dangerous to you as a diabetic because they destroy tissue painlessly.

7 SOCKS. Wear well-fitting socks, without thick toe seams, made of a material that keeps moisture away from the skin, such as acrylic, cotton or wool

PREVENTION

Daily
Inspection

Daily
Washing

Drying Feet

Moisturizing

Nail Care

Treating
Common
Foot
Problems

Socks

Shoe
Selection
& Care

Foot Exam

Exercise

blends. Wear clean, dry socks and change them daily. The Thorlo sock company has developed a padded sock that has been scientifically studied and has the following scientifically proven properties. Reduction of pressure against the foot. Reduction of blisters typically caused by friction and shear forces and reduction of pain and pressure in patients withrheumatoid arthritis. You can wear socks to bed, even two pairs if your feet are cold, but do not use artificial heat sources such as a heating pad, hot water bottle, heated bricks, an open fireplace, or a radiator to warm your feet. Your foot probably will not warm up and your probably will cause a thermal injury to your foot.

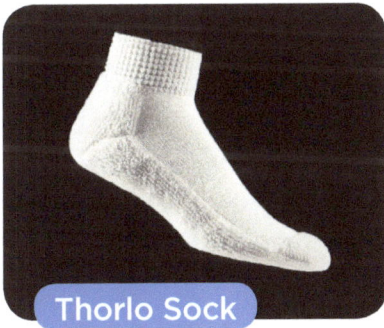

Thorlo Sock

8 **SHOE SELECTION & CARE.** Wear well fitting, soft, leather or fabric shoes or slippers at all times, even at home. Do not wear sandals or open-toed shoes or walk barefoot. Shoes should cover, support, and protect your feet and allow room for your toes to be in their natural posi-

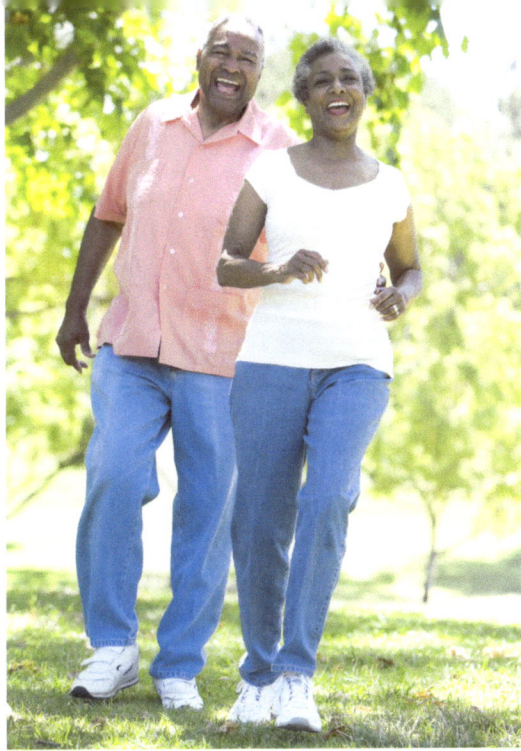

tion. Consult your podiatrist or pedorthist to make sure your shoes fit correctly. Check inside the shoes daily for foreign objects before putting them on.

9 **FOOT EXAM.** When you go to your primary care provider, ask for a foot exam. If you take off your socks and shoes, the doctor will be more likely to look at your feet. To help prevent foot complications, get a foot exam every year that uses a monofilament testing device — an essential diagnostic tool to identify loss of protective sensation for pain, a complication of diabetes. If your foot develops an open wound, a crack in the skin between the toes, or a red, swollen, or locally warm area, you should seek medical attention immediately. Just because you don't feel pain in your feet doesn't mean you don't have a problem.

JUST BECAUSE YOU DON'T FEEL PAIN IN YOUR FEET DOESN'T MEAN YOU DON'T HAVE A PROBLEM.

10 **EXERCISE.** Exercise on a regular basis. Walking and swimming are best. Wear swim sneakers or old tennis shoes to protect your feet from painless injury at the beach or pool.

11 **GET PROPER MEDICAL ATTENTION.** If your foot develops an open wound, a crack in the skin between the toes, or a red, swollen, or locally warm area, you should seek medical attention immediately.

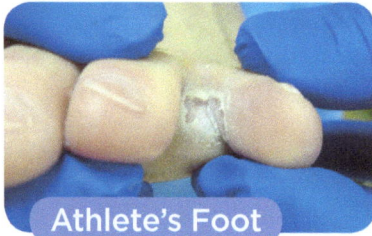
Athlete's Foot

12 **TAKE CARE OF YOUR HEALTH.** Everything your doctor tells you to do to keep your general health and specifically your diabetes under control will also impact your foot health. So, if you keep your blood glucose (sugar), blood pressure, and cholesterol levels in the target range; eat healthy foods, avoid sugary and alcoholic beverages, do not smoke or use tobacco products, limit fat and high caloric intake; exercise thirty minutes a day, at least five days a week; educate yourself about diabetes and practice preventive foot heath behaviors, your feet will also benefit.

2

Basic Foot Hygiene: Washing Your Feet

TOP TIPS

Do's

- Make sure the water temperature isn't too hot by checking it with your elbow.
- Use soap with moisturizer for dry skin. Rinse well.
- Gently pat your feet dry with a soft, fluffy towel, especially between your toes.
- Moisturize dry skin to prevent itching and cracking, especially after a bath or shower.

Don'ts

- Do not soak your feet.
- Do not use lotions with alcohol.
- Do not apply moisturizer between your toes.

Washing Feet With Soap

At the very core of good foot care and good foot health is keeping your feet clean. Your best bet is washing them in a tub or in the shower, but you can use a pan of water or a special foot bath. To keep yourself steady, consider getting a bench for your shower or tub or installing grab bars in your shower. Rinse your feet before you stand up to avoid slipping.

To help you reach your feet, you can purchase a long-handled bath brush or a sponge on a handle.

It's not necessary to soak your feet. In fact, soaking could open small cracks in your skin where germs could get in, and that's where infections start. Soaking may also remove natural skin oils. And repeated wetting and drying actually worsens your dry skin problems.

When choosing soap, look for one that is not milled, it does a better job at moisturizing your skin, because the glycerin is not removed.

Keep your bathing area clean. Bleach can clean areas in the home environment that may be contaminated with bacteria, mold, yeast, or fungus.

Temperature Testing

It is always good to test the water temperature before stepping into a bath or shower. In addition to using your elbow, you can use a bath thermometer. A product called ScaldSafe™ is a floating disc that you can drop into the bath or hold under running water to test the temperature for safety. The disc color will change indicating whether the water is too hot, or the perfect 93.2 degrees Fahrenheit.

Drying Feet

Leave one end of the towel on the floor and rub your foot over the towel to dry it. Dry as well as you can between your toes. Dry feet are as important as clean feet because damp feet can contribute to infections. Even if you are unable to reach your feet or bring your feet up to clean them, you must make an extra effort to be sure to dry them, as well, especially between the toes if you are at risk for foot infections and ulcers.

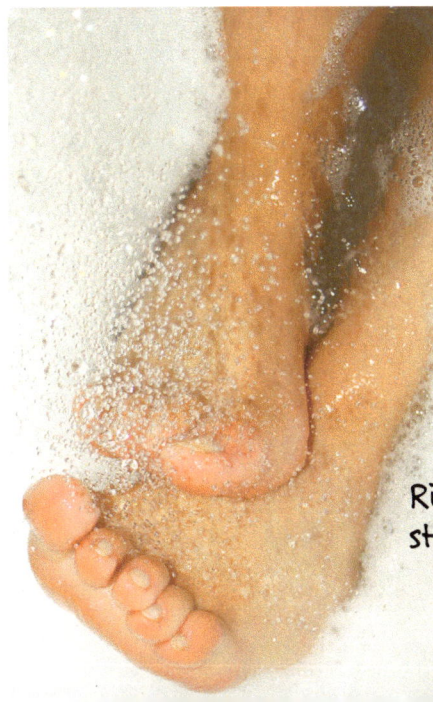

Rinse your feet before you stand up to avoid slipping.

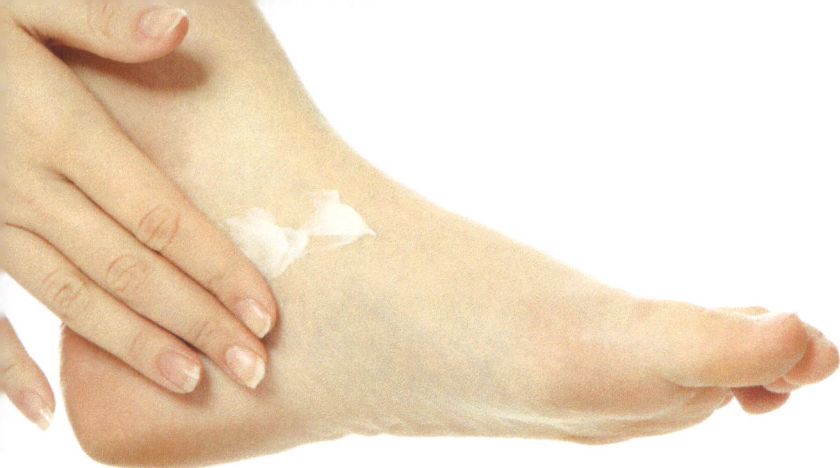

Moisturizing Feet

After a bath or shower is the best time to apply a moisturizer, it helps seal in the moisture your body has absorbed. If you use a lotion sponge, keep it in a plastic bag. Apply moisturizer at least once a day; if you have severe dry skin, two or three times daily. If you keep your moisturizer in your sock drawer, it might remind you to use it.

The best moisturizers contain olive, almond, jojoba, vegetable oil, or aloe vera. Avoid moisturizers, creams, lotions, ointments, or oils with alcohol; it will evaporate and take moisture from the skin. If you are sensitive to chemicals, avoid

THE BEST MOISTURIZERS CONTAIN OLIVE, ALMOND, JOJOBA VEGETABLE OIL OR ALOE VERA. AVOID MOISTURIZERS, CREAMS, LOTIONS, OINTMENTS, OR OILS WITH ALCOHOL

perfumed or colored lotions. And, if you're allergic to wool, avoid lanolin. Moisturizers with Urea work the best for dry skin as they bring moisture from the deep tissues to the most superficial layers of skin.

If you are bathing before you go to bed and putting lotion on your feet, wear socks to help the moisturizer soak in overnight and to be sure it doesn't get all over your sheets.

CHAPTER 3

YOUR
CAREGIVER

One person caring about
another represents life's
greatest value.

—Jim Rohn

People who have a chronic disease such as diabetes often depend on others to help with their care. A caregiver can be a family member, a friend, a neighbor, a volunteer or a paid health care worker. There are many ways caregivers can help you. Here are a few things caregivers can do to support your foot health.

- Help wash your feet
- Help inspect your feet for signs of problems
- Check your shoes and socks for objects, tears or anything that would cause undue pressure
- Take you to the foot care specialist to advocate for you and listen to instructions
- Purchase supplies needed for good foot care: soap, moisturizers, etc.
- Help plan and prepare meals
- Aid with exercise
- Help with medications
- Help with preventive foot care behaviors
- Be a good listener

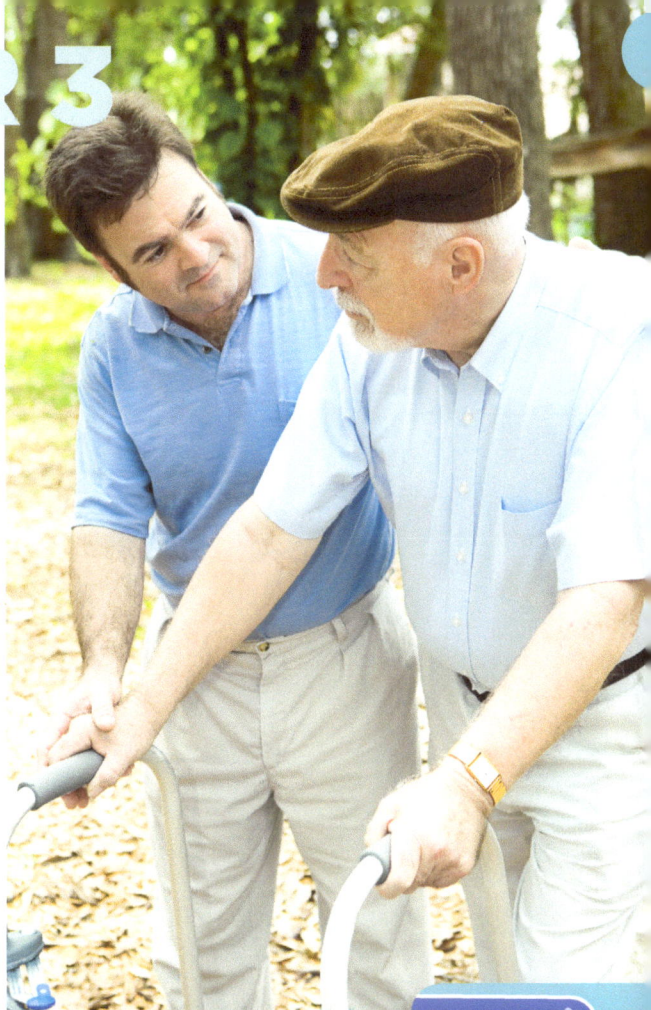

In this chapter

TIPS FOR CAREGIVERS

TOP TIPS For Caregivers

1 TAKE TIME OFF: Separate yourself from this demanding responsibility and do something for yourself every day to help relieve stress and lighten your load.

2 GET HELP: Ask other members of your family to assist

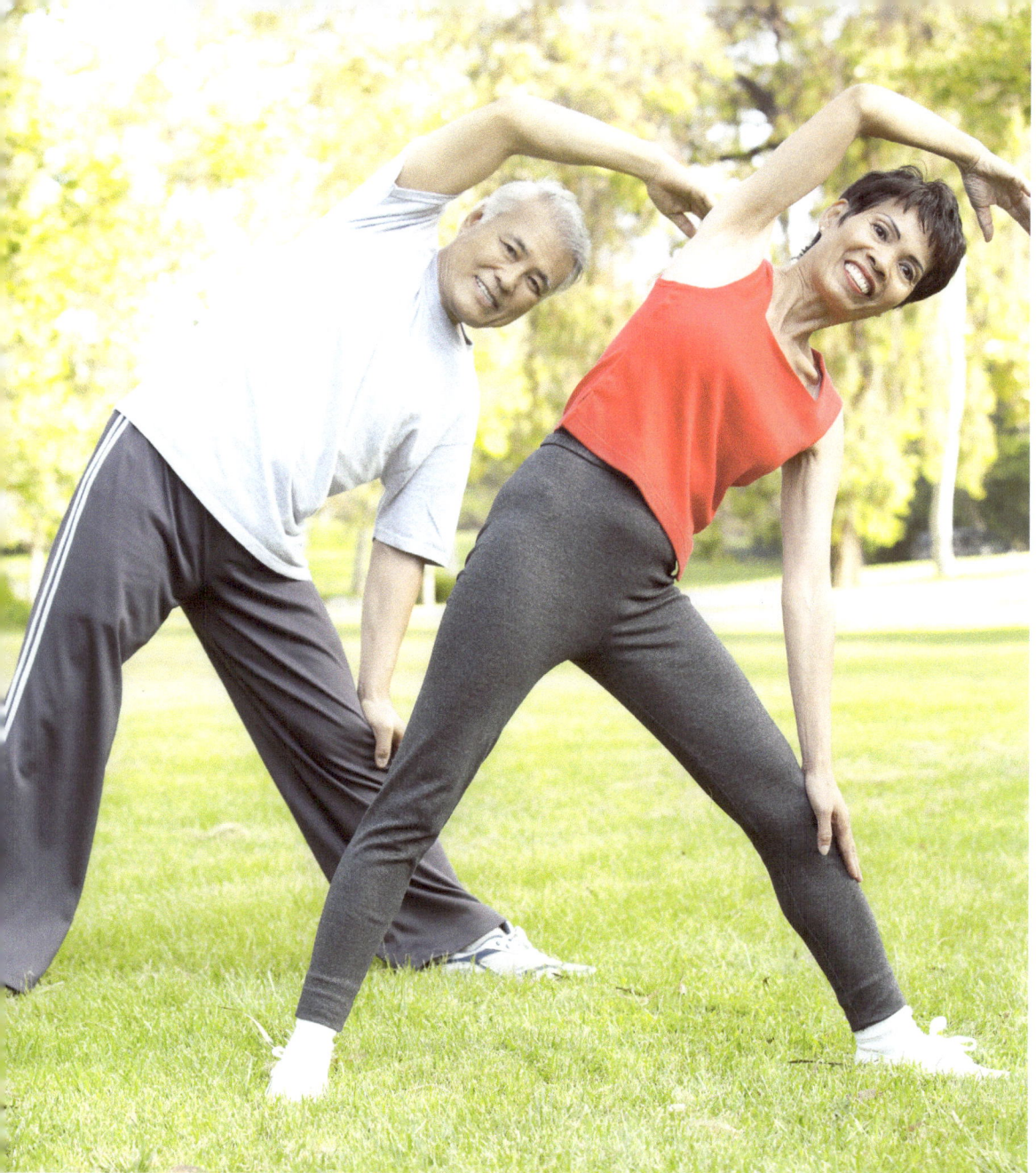

you. Hire someone to help with the chores. Check into services that assist with meal preparation, house cleaning or other jobs you can delegate out.

③ STAY HEALTHY: Get some exercise and make sure you maintain a healthy eating regimen. Keeping your own body in good shape will help you manage your stress level.

④ TALK TO SOMEONE: You may need to vent and get the stress off your shoulders rather than keeping all your thoughts and feelings to yourself. You can talk to a friend, a therapist, or join a caregiver support group.

CHAPTER 4
SELF-CARE

There's only one corner of the universe you can be certain of improving, and that's your own self.

— Aldous Huxley

Y ou must take the major responsibility for your health. Other people and professionals can help you, but only you can control your blood sugars, your eating, your use of tobacco, your exercising, your practicing of preventive foot care behaviors, and your personal hygiene. Yes, we know that this is not easy. Diabetes self-management can be very demanding.

Today, tomorrow, and every day after, you must perform the tasks that will keep your blood sugars as close to non-diabetic normal as possible. There is no vacation. There is little forgiveness for departure from that almighty schedule. And if you lose patience, forget, or give up, it is your health that suffers.

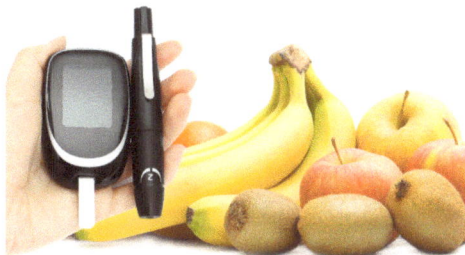

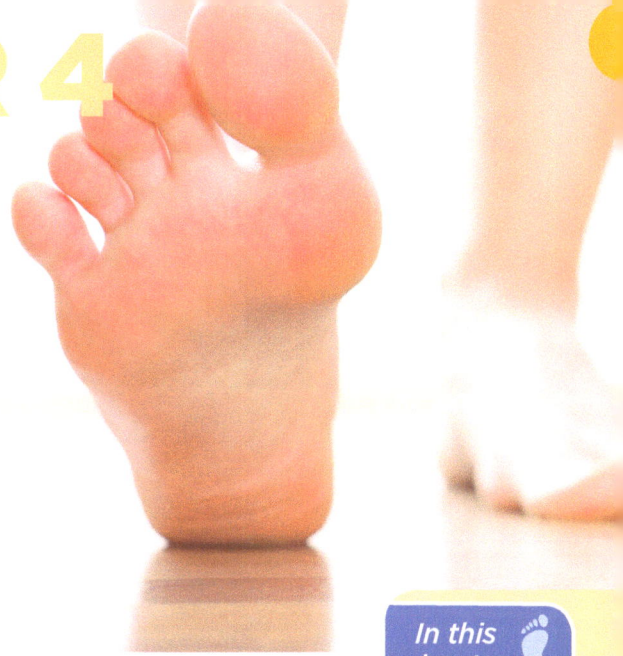

In this chapter

TIPS FOR SELF-CARE

TOP TIPS For Staying on Track

1 HAVE A PLAN & GOALS. Think about and write down your plan for taking care of your diabetes and include your healthcare goals.

2 ASK FOR HELP. You don't have to do it alone. Your diabetes educator can help you make a plan. Your registered dietitian can help you with meal concerns. Talk to the health professionals taking care of you and ask them for help in coming up with solutions to the problems you are facing.

3 INVOLVE FRIENDS AND FAMILY. Share your plan with your friends and family. Ask them to help encourage you. Since taking care of yourself involves adopting healthy habits, ask them to join you in working towards a goal of good health. Consider joining a diabetes support group to share and learn from others with similar issues.

4 EDUCATE YOURSELF.

Get the facts. Understand the options and the consequences. Learn about diabetes. Figure out what you need to do to keep going, and what you can do to make each task easier.

Education

Classes on diabetes have a tremendous benefit in helping you prevent potential problems associated with this disease. Many hospitals have diabetes patient education programs and nutritionists devoted specifically to diabetic care. Don't depend upon your doctor alone to tell you everything you need to know about diabetes and managing the illness with a focus on prevention. It's up to you to educate yourself. With the ever-increasing amount of information available on the Internet and the results of scientific research in this area, take advantage of educational opportunities available online and in your community. See Chapter 20 for a reference list of credible resources online. Help yourself!

Medications

If you are given medication for your foot health, it is important that you follow directions on taking that medication. The Federal Drug Administration (FDA) encourages people to know the following about any medication they are taking:

- The medication's name, strength, daily dosage, and how often it should be taken.

- The purpose of the medication.

- The importance of refills and avoiding lapses in doses.

Create A Partnership

Be partners with all of your health care providers. Each of you has responsibilities and when you work together you have a winning team for your foot health. Remember that only you can do what is necessary to maintain your overall health and your foot health. While no one can guarantee that you will still not have complications, when you do the right things for your health and you do have an issue, it will likely be easier for your medical team to do something for you to alleviate the situation or problem. That is, their treatments will probably work better and faster because you have kept yourself and your feet in good health.

BE PARTNERS WITH ALL OF YOUR HEALTH CARE PROVIDERS.

CHAPTER 5

WALKING & OTHER EXERCISE

Those who think they have no time for bodily exercise will sooner or later have to find time for illness.

— Edward Stanley

The human foot is a complex structure, with more than 40 muscles and tendons, 36 complex joints, 107 ligaments and 26 bones. Together your two feet contain more than 1/4 of all the 206 bones in your body. The foot and ankle together convert a vertical force from our legs into a horizontal force in our feet and allow us to walk, run, jump, dance, and move. The foot is designed to support our weight and to provide balance and mobility. The average person walks 115,000 miles in a lifetime. That is just about three times around the earth!

One of the best ways to keep your muscles, bones and joints young is to stay active. If you have never been active, you can begin slowly, even exercising while you are sitting. Walking is perhaps the healthiest exercise you can do other than swimming. It is good for your heart, brains, bowels, and spirit. Though exercise improves most anyone's health, for people with diabetes, it is even more essential. Exercise improves insulin resistance, increases the circulation, decreases cardiovascular disease, decreases blood sugar levels, and helps control weight, circulation in your legs and feet.

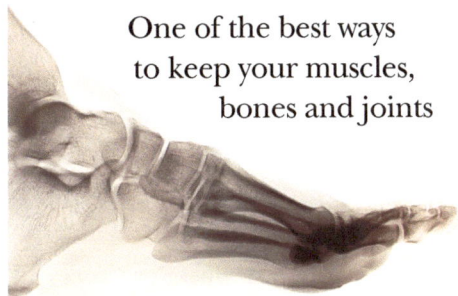

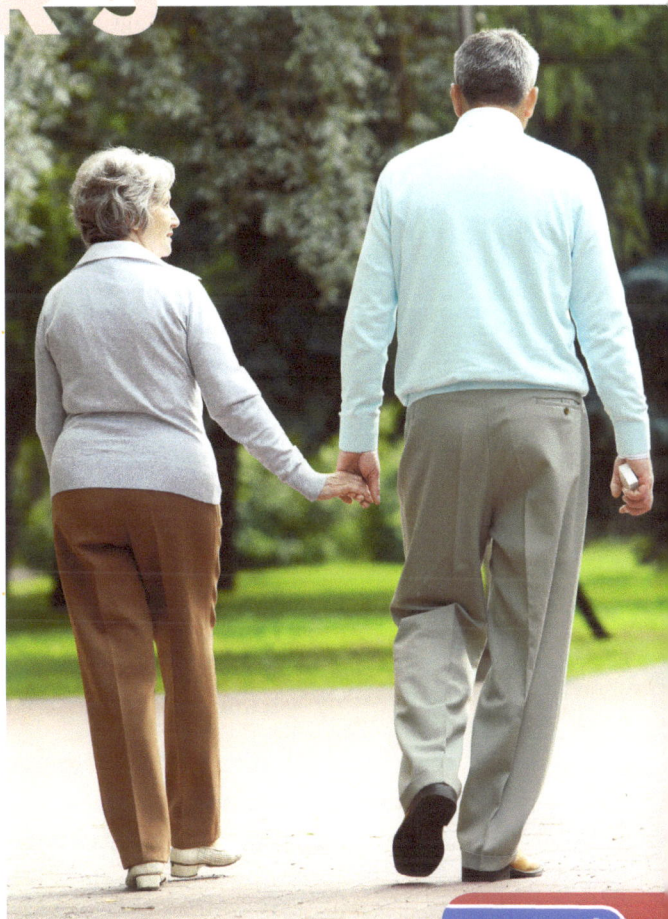

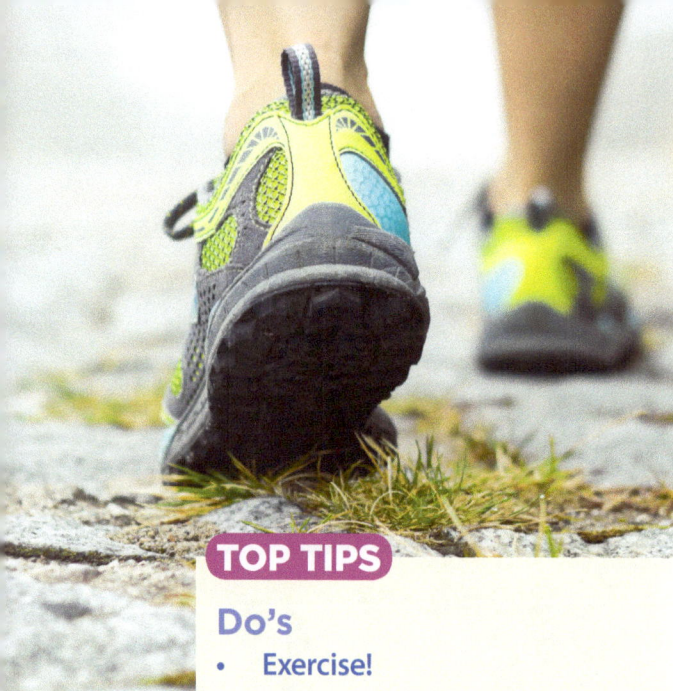

TOP TIPS

Do's

- Exercise!
- Walk (20 minutes/day; twice a day) it can improve your circulation in your legs and feet .
- Drink plenty of water.
- Vary your exercises: aerobics, stretching, strength building.
- Wear good quality athletic shoes for the activity (running shoes, golf shoes, bowling shoes).

Don'ts

- Don't overdo repetitive weight bearing exercises such as jogging and stair climbing if you have loss of protective sensation for pain in your feet.
- Don't do weight-bearing exercises if you have a foot ulcer or loss of protective sensation for pain.
- Don't go barefoot or wear thin-soled sandals or water shoes on hot sand or on pavement.

1 BEFORE EXERCISING

When walking, running, jogging or doing any exercise, it's important for people with diabetes to follow some simple, basic rules:

- Wear clean socks.
- Wear good quality walking or running shoes (or shoes that apply to the sport selected).
- Take time to warm up.
- Stretch slowly.

2 AFTER EXERCISING

- Cool down.
- Stretch.
- Inspect your feet for redness, swelling, blisters, corns or callus buildups.
- If you experience any pain, and are unable to figure out the problem and correct it, see your physician or foot care specialist.

3 TYPES OF EXERCISE

Moving your body is natural and essential for good health. A body is not meant to stay in one position for long periods of time. You need to decide what exercise you can do and how often you can do it. You will more likely stick with a program you enjoy. Consider varying your exercise to keep it interesting and stay motivated. Exercise is a lifetime commitment.

If you have diabetes, check

with your health care provider before you begin an exercise program. Start slowly and gradually increase your endurance. Exercise at least three to four times per week for 20 to 40 minutes each session. It would be ideal if you could find time to exercise every day.

From a foot health care perspective, it is most important that you wear good shoes that are appropriate for the type of exercise you are doing and practice good foot care before and after exercising.

Here are some exercises to consider.

- **Walking, Jogging, Biking, Stair Climbing.** Wear a pedometer to see if you are walking enough. Set your goal for 10,000 steps per day. The average person should walk 4.5 miles per day. Walking gives you the freedom to choose where and when you want to go at your own pace. Walking allows you to freely conduct the affairs of your daily lives without depending on others. Ask any person who has lost a foot or leg and they will tell you, the world is a different place when you lose the ability to walk. Most of us take our feet for granted until something happens that stops our normal function.

ONE STUDY REPORTS THAT AS PEOPLE AGE, THEY BECOME "FEARFUL WALKERS," ADOPTING A SLOWER WALKING SPEED AND SHORTER STRIDE LENGTH.

FACTS

- **Strength building.** Weight lifting, Pilates.
- **Flexibility, Stretching.** Both Yoga and Tai Chi improve glucose metabolism, enhance immune function, lower blood pressure, and aid in weight loss.
- **Swimming.** Swimming is a good exercise, but cold water should be avoided and special protective swim shoes should be worn.

Issues In Walking

• Aging

As you age, your bones can shift out of position. You may lose some of the normal fat pad that cushions the balls of the foot, which may result in calluses. Not having that cushion may make you unsteady and change your gait or walking pattern. When you age, you may lose your sense of balance because of a decrease in the mass of your muscles or atrophy, or due to problems in your inner ear, that involve balance. One study reports that as people age they become "fearful walkers," adopting a slower walking speed and shorter stride length.

• Amputation

People with a below-the-knee amputation must work three times harder to walk with an artificial device that replaces a limb, known as a prosthesis. Those with an above-the-knee amputation exert five times the effort to walk as compared to those of us with all of our original parts.

• Loss of Protective Sensation for Pain

If you can't feel the floor with your feet, you may have trouble walking. This loss of feeling may be due to nerve damage or peripheral sensory neuropathy, a complication of diabetes. You might feel unsteady, trip, or stumble. If you are having trouble with balance, you should check with your physician or foot care specialist. You may benefit from a consultation with a physical therapist who can help you do balance and muscle strengthening exercises, increase your awareness of the position of your feet and perhaps recommend an ankle support, brace or cane. If you do require a cane, the therapist will help you select the right length, an appropriate tip, and help show you how to walk with it.

• Obesity

People who are obese have a different gait from those who are not. Their feet are placed wider than normal because the thighs hold the legs outward. People who are obese often place their body weight more towards the inner part of the foot, which changes the mechanics of walking, putting increased stress on tendons, ligaments and joints.

• Common Foot Problems

If you have structural or bony deformities (such as bunions, tailor's bunions, or toe deformities) or soft tissue deformities (such as corns and calluses), you probably have a biomechanical or functional problem involving how your foot functions when

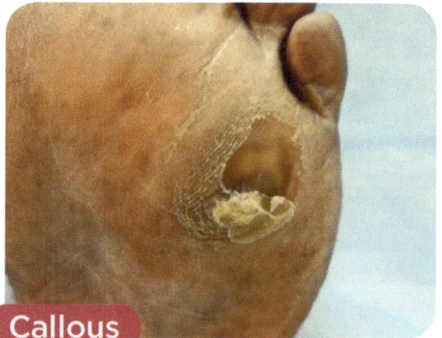

Callous

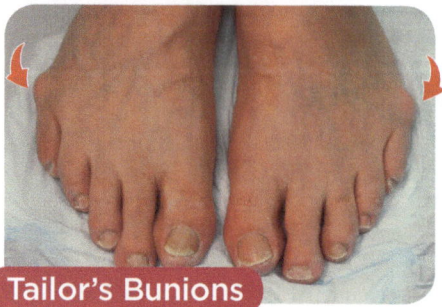

Tailor's Bunions

PEOPLE WITH A BELOW-THE-KNEE AMPUTATION MUST WORK THREE TIMES HARDER TO WALK WITH AN ARTIFICIAL DEVICE THAT REPLACES A LIMB, KNOWN AS A PROSTHESIS.

you walk. Think of it as similar to a misaligned or out-of-balance tire on your car. These problems may cause a loss of balance. Walking with these problems may cause other parts of your body to suffer; thus, you may end up with ankle, knee, hip, or low back pain that may be partly caused by faulty foot mechanics and function.

In the foot, most everyone has two small accessory sesamoid bones located within the long flexor tendon that runs under the first metatarsal, the bone just behind the big toe (hallux). Sesamoid bones are part of a sophisticated system of natural pulleys and levers to provide your muscles with mechanical advantages to function. They provide a mechanical advantage for your big toe with the power to propel you forward in the push-off phase of gait. While they can greatly benefit your ability to walk, they also can be the source of pain, functional disability and the secret cause of foot ulcers under and just behind the big toe.

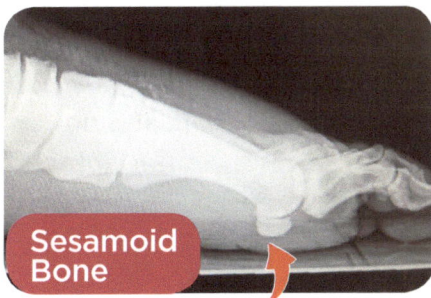

Sesamoid Bone

• Medications

Because of your health issues, you may be taking medications. Every medication has the potential for an adverse side effect. It is not unusual for medications to cause dizziness or lightheadedness. Podiatrists are able to identify people who have a higher risk of falling by watching and analyzing their gait.

• Biomechanics

Biomechanics is the science that studies the relationship of foot structure to foot function. Faulty biomechanical function is one of the keys to understanding why the foot of the person with diabetes may develop an ulcer. Your yearly foot exam should include a biomechanical evaluation, which should examine the following:

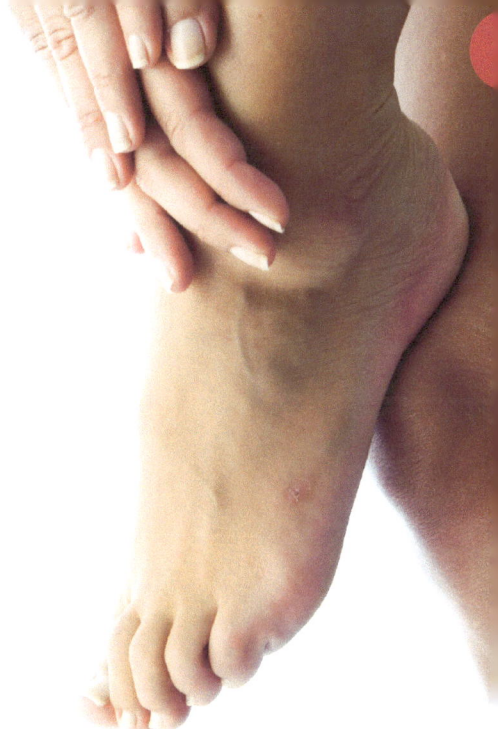

- Joints for their range of motion, pain or limitations of motion.

- The foot's position relative to the floor. Is it in the neutral position or tilted inward or outward?

- The muscle strength of your feet and legs.

- The position of the first metatarsal bone: is it higher or lower than the normal position?

- The length of each of your legs, called limb length. People who have had hip or knee implant surgery often have one leg longer or shorter as a result of the surgery and that difference may contribute to a diabetic foot problem.

After a biomechanical foot examination, you should have a gait analysis. The manner or pattern in which a person walks is called his or her "gait." Scientists refer to the complex musculoskeletal events that occur when you walk as the "gait cycle." The gait cycle includes: contact, midstance, and propulsive phases. When everything goes right, you get from here to there without even thinking about it. When things don't go right, you can develop foot, leg, and even low back problems. Your foot health care specialist understands the relationship between gait and ambulation — the ability to move — and foot biomechanics and how these three affect each other and your foot health. Abnormal functioning may cause you to develop ulcers or other foot health issues. Foot function is influenced by a series of factors that include:

- The size, shape, position, and condition of foot bones and joints they form.

- The normal functioning of the circulation, nerves, and musculoskeletal systems.

- The surface on which you are standing.

- The speed at which you are moving.

- The type of footgear you are wearing.

Why do some people develop foot deformities and have pain while others do not? The answer probably lies in the biomechanics of foot functioning. Your podiatrist can help you identify and treat biomechanical problems using special custom-made shoe inserts call orthotics so that you can walk and do other exercises comfortably and without negatively impacting your foot health.

CHAPTER 6

SOCKS

One can never have enough socks.

—J.K. Rowling

TOP TIPS

Do's

- Always wear socks when you wear shoes.

- If your feet or socks get wet during the day, change socks more often.

- Select socks with breathable fibers, such as cotton or wool, that are blended with acrylic or synthetic material that wicks moisture away from your skin.

- Choose socks without seams.

- Wear socks that are shaped like your feet.

- Change into clean socks daily (more often if you have sweaty feet).

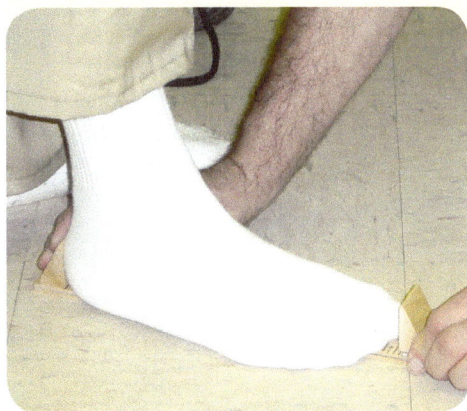

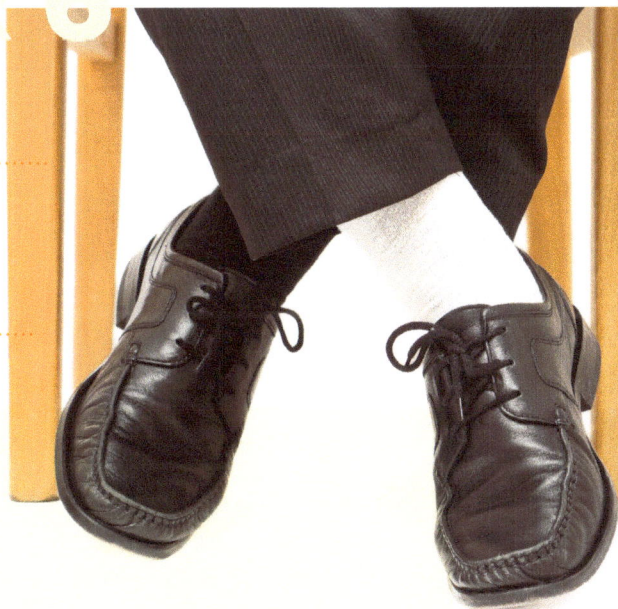

Don'ts

- Don't wear socks that are too loose or too tight; they should fit without folds or wrinkles.

- Don't wear socks with garters, socks that bind, socks with elastic at the top, or socks that fit too tight (you may cut off the circulation to your feet and legs).

- Don't wear socks with holes and don't repair them (rough patches may irritate your foot).

- Don't wear nylon stockings or panty hose (nylon is not a breathable fabric; if you must wear stockings, wear them for a short time only).

In this chapter

DO'S & DON'TS

BEST TYPE OF SOCKS TO WEAR

Choose socks that are shaped like your feet.

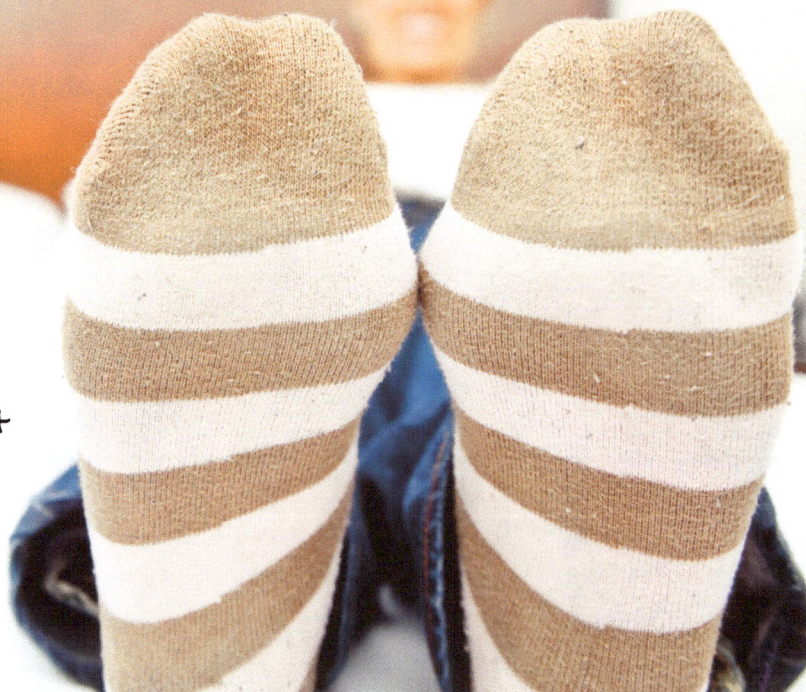

✓

SOCKS

Clean, dry, well-fitting

No seams

Synthetic fibers, latex-free

Minimal or no elastic

① CLEAN DRY SOCKS

Something as simple as wearing clean, dry, well-fitting socks can make a big difference in the health of your feet.

Socks are also important to preventing corns, calluses and blisters that can form next to bunions or digital deformities. Socks can prevent mechanical trauma from shoes that could result in infections, because they act as a protective barrier between the shoe and your foot.

First and foremost, socks must be clean and dry. Bacteria grow well in a warm, dark, damp environment. Clean, dry socks made with the appropriate fibers can help take moisture away from the foot, thus reducing the likelihood of infections. Bleach should be used to clean socks. You can use chlorine or color-safe bleach. If socks begin to show signs of wear, replace them.

② SEAMS

The smartest, safest choice when it comes to protecting your feet is wearing the right type of socks. Any ridge, seam or wrinkle can cause pressure points on the bottom or sides of the foot. Your socks should protect your feet from irritation, discomfort and ulceration that seam edges can cause. Toe seams in socks, for example, can increase pressure on the toes that may cause blisters. People with diabetes who have loss of protective sensation for pain in their feet are at the greatest risk because they cannot feel blisters or cuts (abrasions) as they are developing. All socks have seams somewhere; even tube socks have a seam at the toe. Specialty companies have designed socks with special features for the person with diabetes who is at-risk. These include seams that are flat and non-irritating.

3 FIBERS

You might think that cotton or wool socks would provide the best protection for your feet, but that is not the case. Cotton and wool do absorb moisture, which is important. However, they keep the moisture they absorb right next to your foot. Additionally, these fibers can be abrasive and cause blisters.

Instead, synthetic fibers are a better choice. Hi-bulk acrylic and stretch nylon socks draw moisture away from the skin, where it can evaporate. These fibers are also less prone to wrinkling on the bottom of the foot.

Select latex-free fibers that contain no harmful dyes or additives. Some socks may be dyed with colors that cause people to break out with allergic reactions. Therefore, people with diabetes who are sensitive to color dyes should wear white socks to eliminate this potential problem.

IMPROPERLY FITTED SOCKS, OR A POOR QUALITY KNIT, CAN TRIGGER A FOOT ULCER.

FACTS

4 ELASTIC

Ideally, you want to wear socks that do not have elastic or have only minimal elastic at the top. Elastic can decrease circulation. There are some stretchy, non-binding socks on the market that create uniform compression that actually promote blood flow. Since circulation is always a concern for people with diabetes, these non-elastic socks are a safe choice.

5 DIABETIC SOCKS

Socks may seem rather insignificant in the big picture of preventing foot ulcers and amputations, but they are actually very significant. Improperly fitted socks, or a poor quality knit can trigger a foot ulcer. One of the several brands of socks on the market for people with diabetes is SensiFoot™. Their website says that they use an acrylic, multi-fiber blended knit, which offers greater protection because it wicks moisture away from the skin to the outer surface where it can evaporate. SensiFoot™ socks are made specifically for people with diabetes or arthritis. They combine comfort and protection with an antifungal and antibacterial finish, and are machine washable.

6 COMPRESSION STOCKINGS

Compression stockings are used to keep fluid from collecting in the legs and to limit swelling (edema). These stockings are graded by the amount of pressure or compression they exert against the skin: mild, moderate or high. Wearing the wrong size stocking can be uncomfortable. You should measure around your calf at the widest part and from the floor to your knee to get the right size. It is also important that the stockings are not too loose or too tight. Custom fittings are available as well as zippered stockings. There are below-the-knee or above-the-knee styles.

Compression stockings can be difficult to put on and to take off. It is best to put them on in the morning, before your feet or ankles swell. There is an aid called a stocking butler that can help.

People with poor circulation, skin disorders, infections, open wounds or massive swelling should NOT wear support hose. DO NOT wear support hose to bed.

7 OTHER SPECIAL SOCKS

Foot Odor

Bacteria on the foot usually causes foot odor and that possibility should be investigated and treated. There are socks designed to help control foot odor available in large drugstores or from a podiatrist. (Foot odor may also be contained with special insoles with activated charcoal.)

Sizes

Big and Tall shops often have extra-large sized socks.

Sweat

Sport stores now have two or three-layered socks designed to better absorb sweat. Some are double knit on the bottom with an extra layer of cushioning. There are new socks on the market with copper that is blended into the threads to reduce perspiration and decrease bacterial and fungal infections. (www.cupronsales.com)

DO NOT

WEAR SUPPORT HOSE TO BED

CHAPTER 7
SHOES

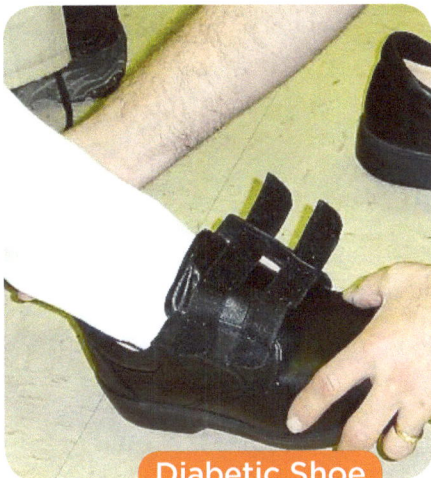

> I cried because I had no shoes. Then I met a man who had no feet.
>
> — Wally Lamb

When you have diabetes, it is crucial that you use shoes that fit well and are comfortable. Shoes cover, support, and protect your feet. Properly fitted and well maintained shoes can help prevent foot problems. On the other hand, shoes that do not fit correctly can contribute to or exacerbate existing foot health issues. On the bright side, if you've been having foot issues, sometimes, just finding the proper fitting shoe is all it takes to make you feel better.

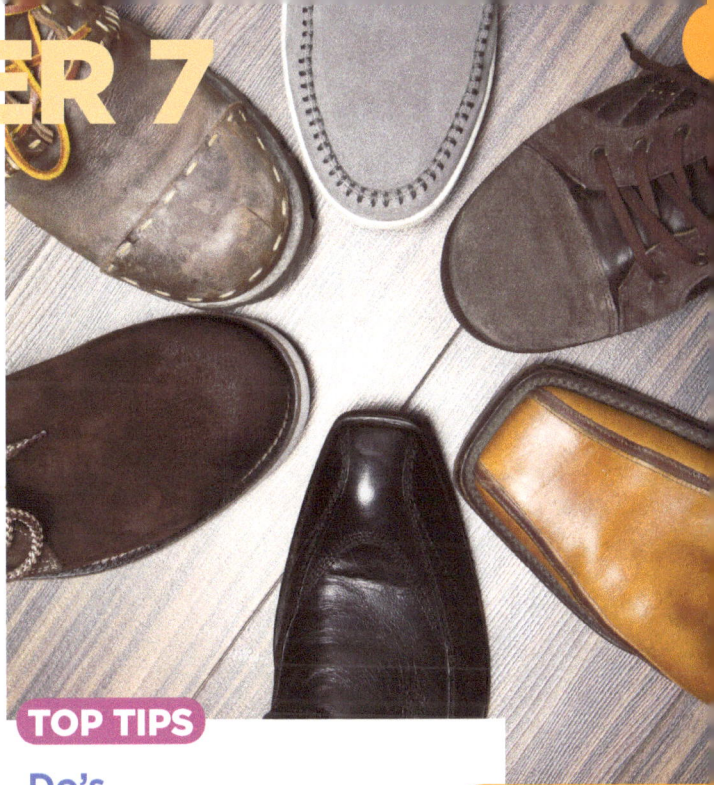

Diabetic Shoe

TOP TIPS

Do's

- Buy shoes that fit comfortably, immediately. Measure both feet and fit the larger foot.

- Check feet more carefully and frequently when wearing new shoes.

- Wear shoes that allow air to circulate (Choose shoes made of natural fibers such as leather or fabric that breathes).

- Allow your shoes to dry out between wearing. Shoes absorb perspiration.

- Look for a shoe that is shaped like a foot .

- Wear protective footwear at a beach or pool (avoid exposure to virus, bacteria, or foreign bodies and foot injuries).

In this chapter

DO'S & DON'TS

BEST SHOES

BUYING SHOES

CUSTOM OR MODIFIED SHOES

INSOLES

PEDORTHISTS

ORTHOTICS

Do's

- If your feet are numb or if you have sensory neuropathy, keep your shoes on all of the time. The only time you may take off your shoes is when you go to bed or when you bathe. Wear house shoes or slippers when at home ONLY if they support, cover, and protect your feet.

- Inspect your shoes every day; look for anything that might injure your feet, like a foreign body, a ripped lining or a defect in the insole.

Don'ts

- Don't go barefooted or sock-footed, EVER, even at home. Your home may be the most dangerous place to walk without shoes because you may have a false sense of security at home. Yet, you can easily injure your foot by stepping on a pin, a tack, a piece of glass or an insulin needle. Be especially cautious when walking on carpeting, as there may be an object hidden in the carpet that can trip you or injure your foot. You may even injure your foot by bumping it against a piece of furniture or a doorframe.

- Don't wear open-toed shoes: clogs, thongs, sandals or flip-flops.

- Don't wear plastic or synthetic shoes.

- Avoid tight, pointed shoes.

- Avoid high heels; they force the weight of the body onto the front of the foot that can jam the toes, increase pressure on the front of your foot, and cause corns, calluses, and ulcers.

- Don't wear shoes you've saved for years for special occasions.

- Avoid walking in the rain or snow.

BEST SHOES FOR PEOPLE WITH DIABETES

- Good quality athletic shoes
- Walking shoes
- Lace-up or velcro closure shoes with a high, rounded toe box
- Diabetic shoes or extra depth shoes
- Custom molded shoes

HOUSE SHOES

You do need to wear shoes even if you are home because you can still step on a sharp object, an object can fall on your foot, or you may bump your foot against a doorframe, table or chair. If you choose to wear a house shoe or slipper, be sure it will provide enough protection to prevent an injury to your foot.

HELPFUL DEVICES

- Shoes with Velcro fasteners are

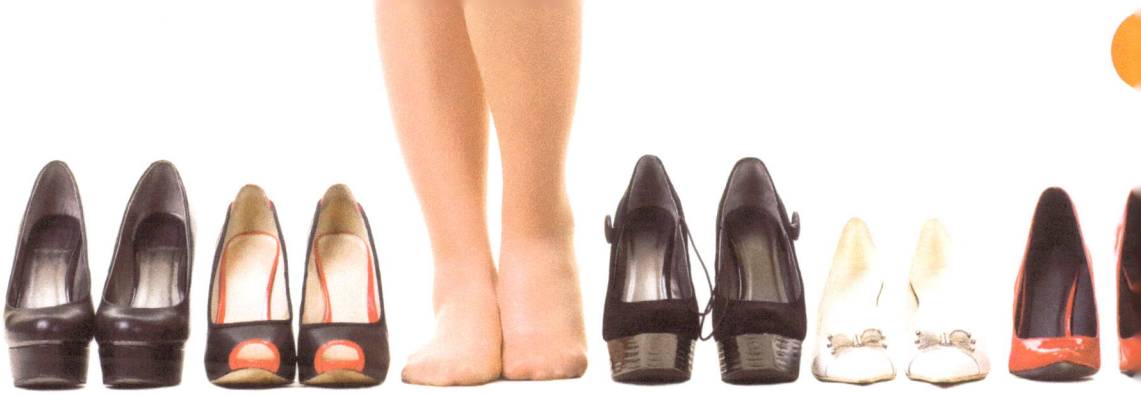

easier to slip on if you have trouble reaching your feet, tying your shoelaces of if you have arthritis.

- Elastic laces found in shoe repair shops make it easier to get shoes on and off without lacing and can enhance the fit.

- Long-handed shoehorns help in slipping shoes on when you can't reach down.

BUYING SHOES THAT FIT CORRECTLY

Here are some tips for buying shoes for people with diabetes:

1 **SHOE SIZE:** Use the shoe size only as a guide. Your shoe size may change as you get older, and the shoe industry's measuring guides have changed over the past twenty years as well. Do not rely on a size that you may have been wearing for years. Have both your feet measured and fit the larger foot. Very few people have the exact same size on both feet. Do not rely on the size of the shoe to be the proper fit for your foot. European and Asian-made shoes have a totally different system of sizing shoes. Try tracing your foot, cutting out the paper and placing it on the sole of the shoe. See whether the shape of the shoe matches the shape of your foot. It is not recommended that you buy shoes online. There is no substitute for trying on your shoes. If you have diabetes and loss of protective sensation for pain or peripheral sensory neuropathy in your feet, you may find it more difficult to get a "comfortable" fitting shoe. Since your foot may be partially or totally numb, you will have difficulty feeling if the shoe fits right and might tend to buy shoes that are a bit too tight, because then you can feel the shoe.

2 **BUYING TIME:** Buy shoes late in the day. Gravity pulls fluid down toward our feet and as the day progresses, there is likely to be more fluid collecting towards the feet and ankles. Shoes bought late in the day will be comfortable all day. Shoes bought in the morning may well be uncomfortable by days' end.

3 **SOCKS:** Wear the appropriate type sock or stocking for the shoe you are buying.

4 INSOLES/SUPPORTS:
If you wear an arch support, accommodative insoles, or prescription custom biomechanical orthotics, bring them with you while shoe shopping so you can "test" them in the shoe store.

5 COMFORT: Be sure the shoes fit comfortably immediately. There is no such thing as taking them home and breaking them in.

6 MATERIALS: Buy shoes constructed from natural materials, such as leather or other natural fibers. Natural materials permit the foot to "breathe," that is, to dissipate heat and perspiration. The uppers or top portion of the shoes should be made of natural materials and should have an adequate sole for shock absorption and protection of the foot.

7 CLOSURES: Consider alternative closures if you have arthritis or any difficulty using shoe laces. There are variations on lacing shoes, such as elastic laces, that can change the pressure against your foot, make it more comfortable and allow you to get shoes off and on without untying and tying laces. For definitive information on shoe lacing, visit www.fieggen.com/shoelace/lacingmethods.htm. Velcro closures are another good option.

8 SUPPLY: Have several pairs of comfortable shoes so that you can alternate what you wear.

9 ACTIVITY: If you are an active adult who enjoys golf, bowling, ice skating, working, skiing, horseback riding, dancing and going out, you will need to purchase several different pairs of shoes for different activities. The shoes you wear throughout the day can vary according to your activities. As for dress shoes, it is strongly recommended that you do not wear high heels. However, if you must wear them for a special occasion, wear the lowest heel possible for the shortest time possible. Make sure they fit well and bring a comfortable pair of shoes into which you can change.

10 FOOT MEASUREMENT:
Make sure your foot is properly measured. The Ritz Stick and Brannock device are the two most common types of measuring devices. In addition to measuring length and width, the Brannock measures heel-to-ball length. This is a relative measurement of the length of your arch to the overall length of the foot. It is helpful to take into account the circumference or volume of your foot, because it can determine the appropriate heel height, toe box shape, and volume of the finished

shoe. If you have two different sized feet, or only one foot, you can contact the National Odd Shoe Exchange, (www.oddshoe.org) which can match you with another member who has the opposite problem.

DAILY CHECKING OF SHOES

1. Look over the uppers, the heels and soles of your shoes for defects.

2. Shake out your shoe and be sure there are no objects like keys, coins or other things that could injure your foot.

3. Run your hand into and over the shoe. You are checking for:

- Cracked uppers or rough seams which could rub a blister
- Worn or loose linings
- Pebbles, coins, keys, foreign objects, or other debris
- Nails or tacks through the sole

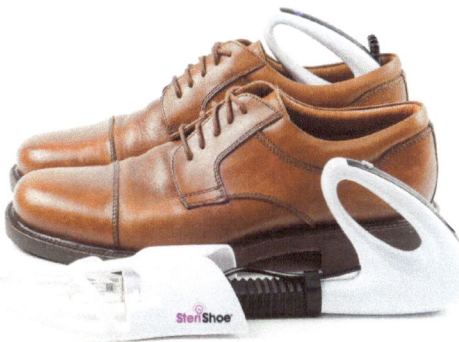

SteriShoe Sanitizer

If you have two different sized feet, or only one foot, contact the National Odd Shoe Exchange, (oddshoe.org) to match you with another member who has the opposite problem.

FACTS

- Signs of the heels or soles wearing down
- A 21st Century method to disinfect your shoes is with the SteriShoe Sanitizer. Scientific research has proven that the SteriShoe ultraviolet shoe sanitizer was shown to be effective in reducing the amount of bacteria and fungus in shoes. (www.sterishoe.com.)

CHANGE YOUR SHOES AS YOUR FEET AGE

Even as an adult, you may not always wear the same shoe size. As people age, their feet tend to get longer, wider, and flatter. You can offset some of the effects of aging by always wearing shoes that fit well. Since changes in the shape of your foot are gradual, you may not realize that your shoes fit poorly, especially if you have nerve damage and can't feel your feet.

GETTING A PRESCRIPTION FOR CUSTOM OR MODIFIED SHOES

Today, there is a wide array of shoes in various widths and depths that can accommodate insoles or orthotics or that can be modified to meet special needs. Shoes can be altered to create custom closures or soles. Before you go through the expense of a custom-made shoe, ask whether a modification of a standard shoe could meet your needs.

If you have any of the following, you may want to consider getting modifications or ordering a custom-made shoe.

- Severe foot deformity
- Bony deformities such as a bunion or digital deformities
- Risk of amputation
- Toe or partial foot amputation
- An ulcer, even if it is now healed
- A history of diabetic-related foot problems
- A wider front of the foot and narrower back
- Feet that are changing shape or losing feeling

✓

TIPS FOR BUYING SHOES

Shoe size

Buying time

Socks

Insoles/ Supports

Comfort

Materials

Closures

Supply

Activity

Foot Measurement

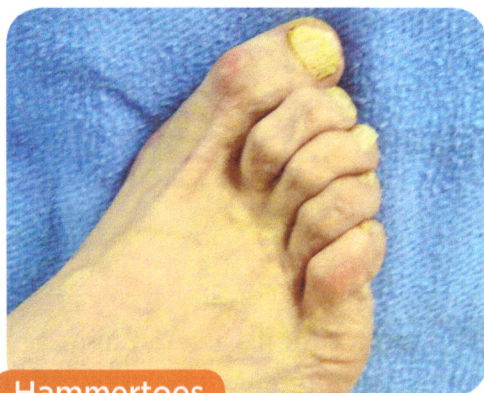

Hammertoes

- Loss of the protective fat pad on the bottom of your foot
- Rheumatoid arthritis that impacts your feet
- Limited range of motion in the joints
- Pain when walking with standard footwear
- Problems in the way the foot functions

SURGICAL SHOES

If you have a foot infection, you should not wear the shoe that you wear everyday; you should wear a surgical shoe. Everyday footwear that has a closed toe box can create an environment that is warm, dark, and moist, which encourages the growth of bacteria, mold, yeast, and fungus and can worsen your foot infection. Surgical shoes cover, support, and protect the foot while providing an environment conducive to healing a foot wound. They can also accommodate bandages or dressings that will not fit into regular footwear. Surgical shoes have a flexible sole with nylon uppers and Velcro™ closures.

EXTRA-DEPTH SHOES

If you have a bunion or a hammertoe, you may need shoes that are extra wide or extra deep. The extra-depth shoe is one-quarter to three-eighths of an inch deeper than the average shoe. This provides room for either custom-made insoles like biomechanical orthotics or over-the-counter inserts. They can also accommodate mild to moderately deformed feet caused by bunions or digital deformities. If you have partial loss of muscular function of your legs due to diabetic motor neuropathy, low back problems, or other medical conditions, you may have difficulty walking, trip over your own feet, and have a high risk of falling in standard shoes. These shoes can also accommodate braces that may be worn for a complication of diabetes called drop foot.

DIABETIC SHOES

It is critical that you have both feet measured and receive proper fitting for your diabetic shoes. Diabetic shoes have the ability to be modified to accept a hinged drop foot brace that stabilizes the foot and leg, helps people walk with better function, and reduces the chances of tripping or falling. Diabetic shoes are constructed with an insert (or insole) usually made of multi-density materials with a pink insole section called plastizote that contacts the foot. This material offers a relatively frictionless surface so it can

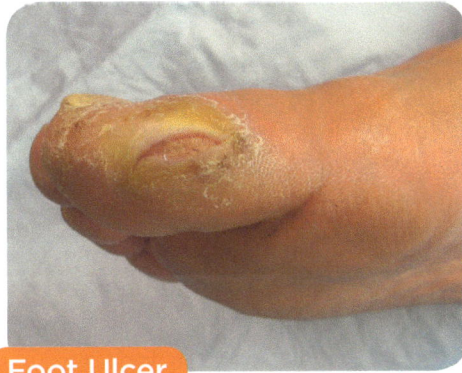

Foot Ulcer

protect your foot from the forces of friction and shear. It also provides a cushioned platform for your foot. One drawback is that it does have the tendency to "bottom out;" that is the material compresses under the sites of the most pressure and loses its ability to protect the foot.

Once plastizote breaks down, the corresponding area of the foot becomes vulnerable to the forces of repetitive microtrauma. Then a protective thickening of skin (a callus) can form on the bottom of the foot. Left untreated, these calluses can lead to abscess or ulcers forming underneath them and can ultimately lead to soft tissue infections, bone infections and amputations.

It's a good idea to write the date on the bottom of the insole when you place it in the shoe so you can monitor how long you have been using it and when it might be time to replace it. A good rule of thumb is to replace the insole about every six months.

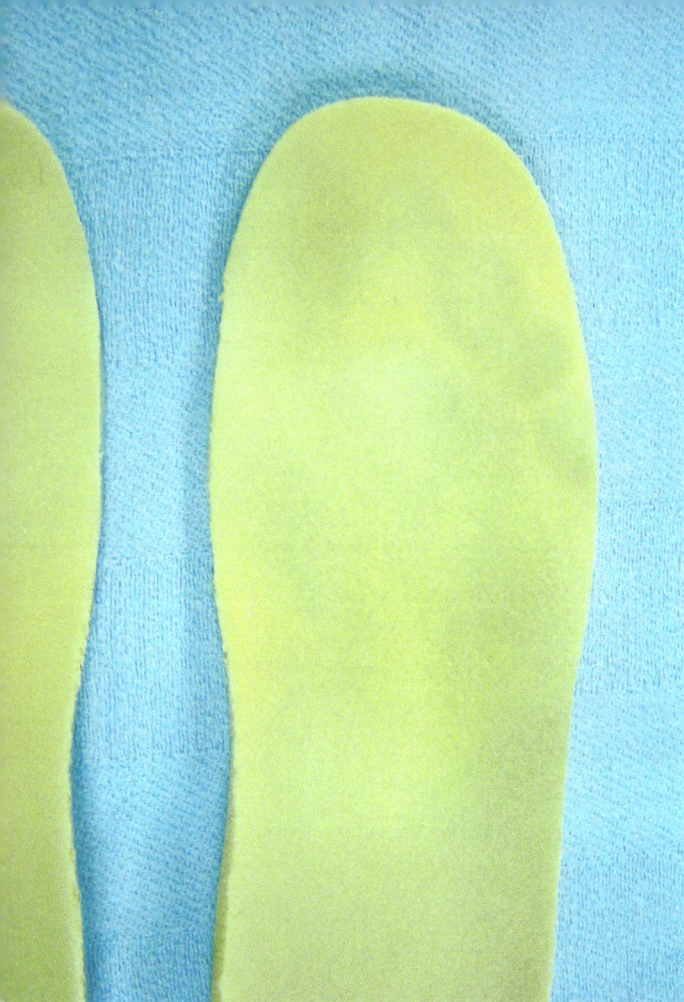

lost mobility to the foot and to relieve or reduce pressure. A rocker sole is applied to the bottom of a normal shoe and permits the shoe to "rock forward" to assist in the push-off phase of gait. It is especially helpful if you have arthritic changes to the big toe joint that prevent normal functioning of the toe when walking.

STILL OTHER MODIFICATIONS

Pieces of steel can be embedded into the sole of your shoe and travel the length of the shoe, making the rocker sole more stable. Stabilization can also involve adding material to a portion of the shoe to stabilize a particular part of the foot. Cushioned heels can be used to add shock absorption for you if your foot has lost its normal fatty tissues in the heel. Wedges help redirect the weight-bearing position of the foot and stabilize a corrected position in a deformity.

CUSTOM-MOLDED SHOES

Custom-molded shoes are made from a cast of your feet. They are prescribed for more extreme cases of deformities, such as bunions, deformed toes or Charcot Foot. They can accommodate specialized insoles like biomechanical orthotics, arch supports or braces and can be modified in style, color, and type of closure.

SOLE MODIFICATION

The outside of the shoe can also be modified. For example, a common exterior modification is rocker soles, used to return

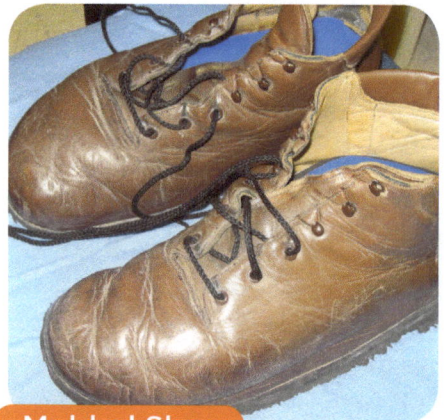

Molded Shoes

Extensions increase the thickness or height of a shoe.

People with diabetes who have had knee or hip joint replacements often have one leg longer than the other after the surgery. This can cause problems with walking and can result in pain in a joint that was previously not painful. Unequal limb length problems can be treated by adding a lift to the sole of the shoe on the shorter limb.

If your foot is wider in the front and narrower in the back, you many need a special type of shoe called a "combination last" shoe. Not all manufacturers make this special type of shoe and, therefore, the styles of shoes that fit you correctly may be limited. If you have identified your foot type as needing this type of shoe, ask for it specifically. New Balance ™ shoes are made in varied widths; this may offer you a better fit.

PEDORTHISTS

Pedorthists are professional shoe fitters who are trained in both foot anatomy and shoe construction. They fill prescriptions for shoes, shoe modifications, insoles, orthotics or braces for footwear. They may work out of a custom shoe store. It is their job to provide the best-fitting footwear for people with foot problems.

TO FIND A PEDORTHIST
GO TO www.abcop.org

If they are certified, you will see the letters C.Ped. after their name. Education for pedorthics started in 1961; since then, podiatry schools have developed pedorthic training programs that prepare individuals for board certification in the field. A board certified pedorthist must pass a comprehensive examination that includes knowledge of anatomy and physiology, pathology and injury, and examination and evaluation of the foot and ankle; footwear and orthotics, including fit, design, construction, materials, modification, adjustment, and follow-up; and management techniques.

Pedorthists understand the anatomy of a shoe, what modifications can be made, and what type of shoe would be best for your foot problem. Ask your pedorthist any questions you may have about proper footwear and fit. After you get your custom-made shoes, you may need to make follow-up visits to be sure that your shoes continue to fit correctly and to serve the purpose for which they were designed.

ORTHOTICS and ARCH SUPPORT INSOLES

If you have foot pain; a thick callus; a change in foot shape that prevents you from walking normally; or knee, hip, or lower back pain caused by faulty bio-mechanics, you may be helped by orthotics.

Orthotics are specially- designed insoles, worn inside your shoes, to control the way your foot moves or to support painful areas of your foot or offload areas of your foot that are vulnerable to ulceration. Orthotics can also be used to prevent recurrent ulcers. They are usually custom-made, using a model of your foot that may be created by a plaster impression, a resin cast, or a computer scan. Some orthotics are made from rigid materials, like carbon fiber, that fully controls movement of the foot. Some are made of plastic that has the ability to both control the foot function and provide shock absorption; others are made from cork and leather, which are softer and more accommodating to your foot. An orthotic is designed to fit the unique shape of your feet, has no artificial elevation of the arch and works in harmony with how nature has designed your foot to function. Medically corrective foot orthotics require a prescription from a health

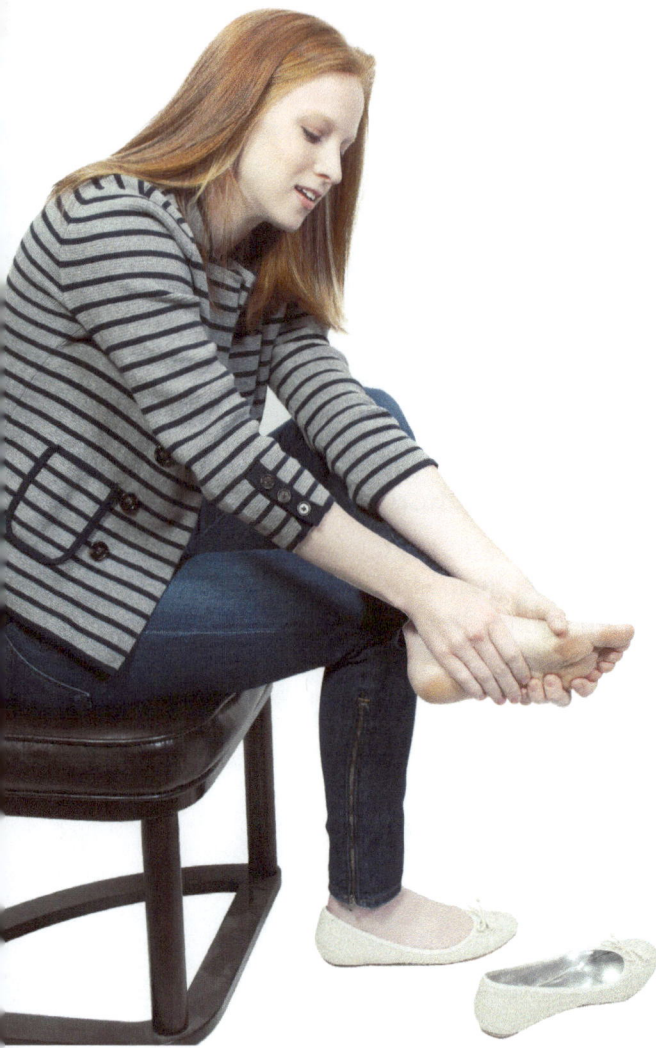

Pedorthics is still a very small profession. There are only about 3,000 Pedorthists in the United States. The best way to find a pedorthist is to go to www.abcop.org and type in your city and state. It will give you the name and contact information for a pedorthist in your neighborhood.

Medicare or insurance may cover prescription footwear, check with your provider. Some major insurance companies now also provide coverage for pedorthic services.

care professional.

Orthotics can help you walk normally; relieve foot pain; help you avoid getting calluses and corns; and may also help relieve foot, knee, hip and lower back pain. You will likely need different orthotics for different shoes and for different activities; and, they should be evaluated and replaced as necessary.

Over-the-counter, mass-produced insoles sold in retail locations are better described as arch supports. They provide an extra cushioning layer between your foot and the floor. If your shoes have thin soles or high-pressure areas where calluses may develop, adding insoles may relieve pressure on your feet. They are often available in drug, grocery or sporting goods stores.

A consideration of wearing an insole or an orthotic is that it will likely take up some room from your shoe; thus, you will likely need more room in the toe box. You can adjust your shoe by removing the original insole that came with your shoe or you can get half length insoles, which don't go under the toes. You should change insoles every three to six months to prevent foot odor and athlete's foot. Magnetic insoles are still controversial; the medical literature has not fully endorsed their use as a treatment for any

YOU SHOULD CHANGE INSOLES EVERY THREE TO SIX MONTHS TO PREVENT FOOT ODOR AND ATHLETE'S FOOT.

specific foot problem.

If you have diabetes, it is likely that over-the-counter insoles will be inadequate for the needs of your feet. The downside of medically-prescribed orthotics; however, is that they can be expensive. In many cases, the value that orthotics provide to the foot is well worth the expense. Check with your health plan to see if it covers orthotics.

Crocs are a 21st century shoe that is made of a heavy duty plastic that covers supports and protects the foot. They have several openings in the shoe to allow for air flow and a strap to secure the shoe around the heel. Crocs are an exception to the rules of foot gear and may safely be used by people with diabetes. Crocs will also accommodate insoles whether they are arch supports or orthotics.

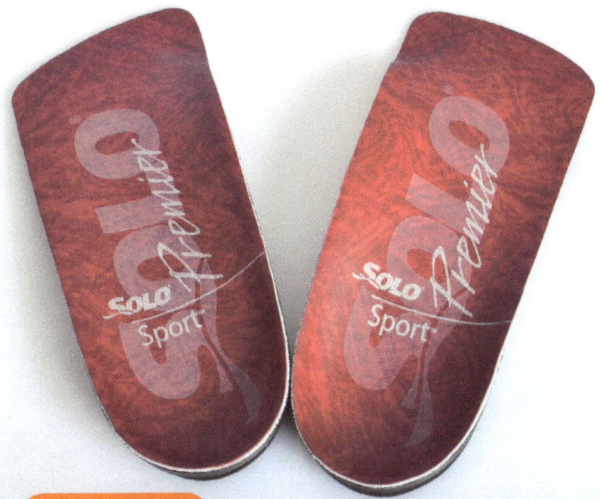

Orthotics

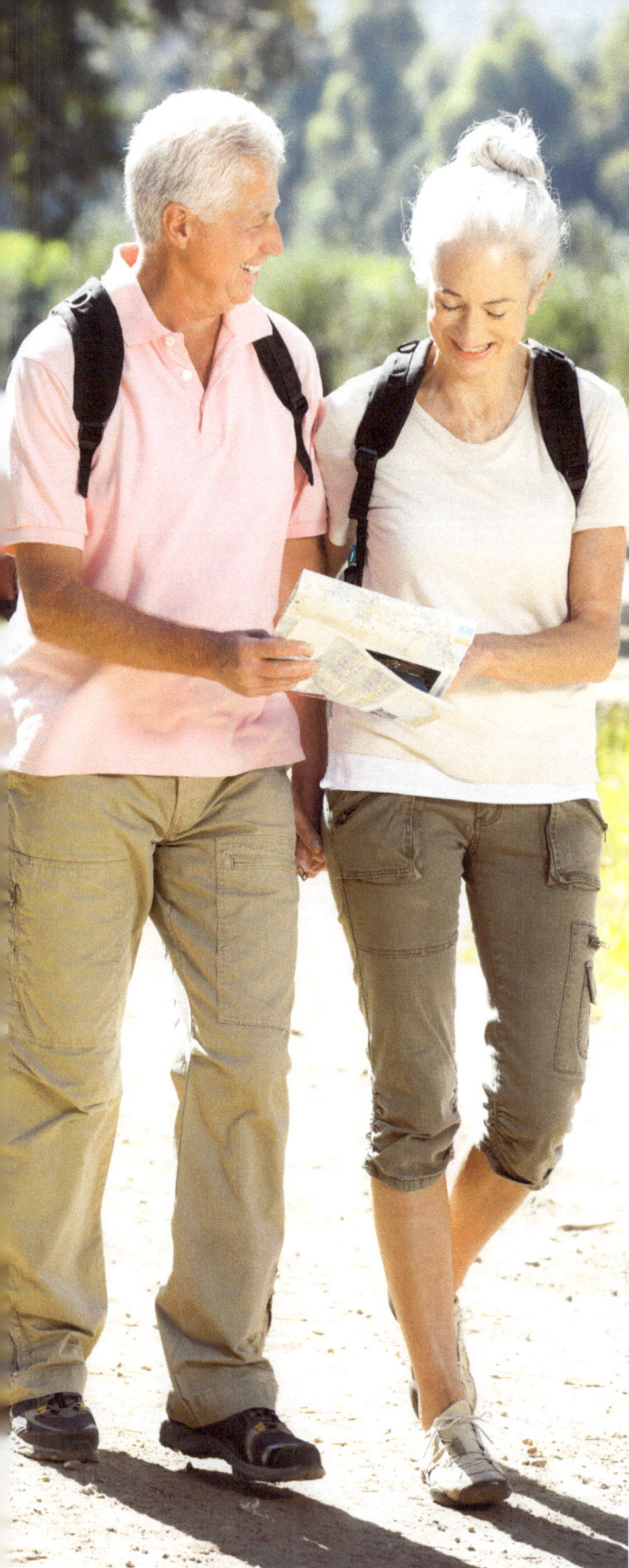

The Crocs Cloud model is suggested for people with diabetes, impaired circulation, impaired sensation, or who have ultra sensitive feet. This shoe is touted to have a super-soft foot bed provides a gentle environment for sensitive feet, while the roomy toe box allows for use of a heavy sock without creating any tightness or pressure points on the foot. The protective front toe cap and elevated heel rim protect the diabetic foot from stubbing and bruising.

ALLOW YOUR
SHOES TO DRY
OUT BETWEEN
WEARING.
SHOES ABSORB
PERSPIRATION.

CHAPTER 8

SKIN

{The largest organ of your body, covering 2 square meters. }

What spirit is so empty and blind, that it cannot recognize the fact that the foot is more noble than the shoe, and skin more beautiful than the garment with which it is clothed?

— Michelangelo

Healthy skin is your main defense against infection. Keeping your skin healthy is the result of a good hygiene, good diet, good maintance and daily inspection.

TOP TIPS

Do's

- Use a moisturizing cream or lotion on your skin from your knees to your toes daily to keep it moist.
- See a foot care specialist if you skin turns colors.
- Ask for help if you can't apply lotion to your feet by yourself.

Don'ts

- Don't put moisturizing lotion between your toes.
- Don't use lotion with alcohol.
- Don't scratch dry skin.
- Don't bathe in very hot water.
- Don't use harsh soaps on dry skin.
- Don't soak your feet.

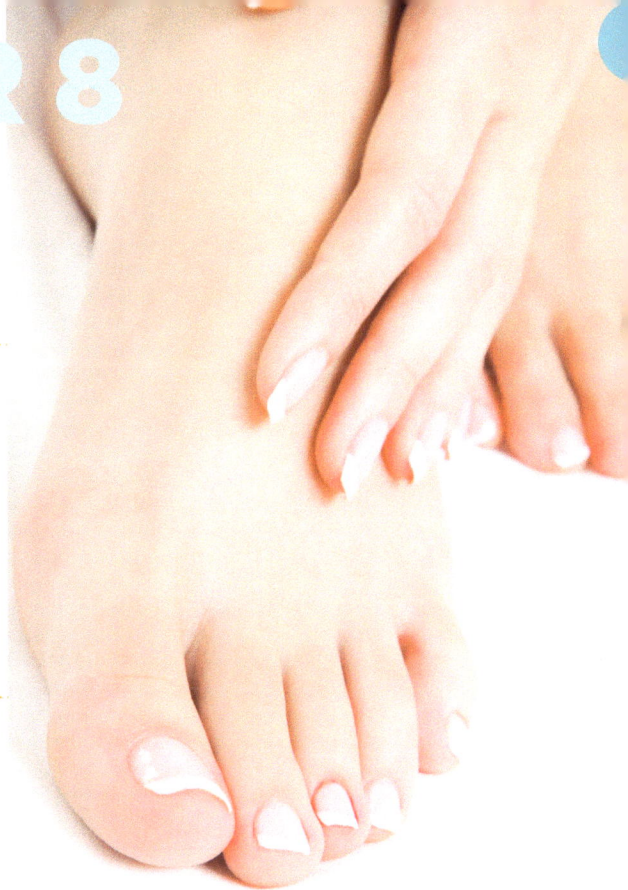

CAUSES OF DRY SKIN

1. Nerve damage, the result of autonomic neuropathy

2. A malfunction of your thyroid gland

3. Aging skin that becomes thinner and dryer

4. Heating systems that blow dry air, commonly used in winter

5. Bathing with very hot water, which washes away natural skin oils

6. Harsh soaps and detergents that also remove these oils

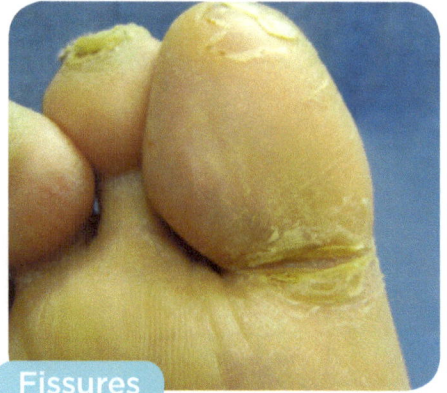
Fissures

NERVE DAMAGE MAY CAUSE DRY SKIN

Dry, cracking skin on your foot is a condition that you should take seriously. There are a variety of medical reasons for dry skin; at the top of the list is nerve damage. This malfunction of the nervous system affects the nerves that support the glands that secrete oil and sweat. When those glands fail to function, the result is dry, flaky skin that seems to affect the entire leg. This can be very itchy and therefore dangerous. Repeatedly scratching this dry skin can lead to an infection and an ulcer on the leg.

One type of nerve damage that is caused by chronically elevated blood sugars is known as Autonomic Neuropathy. The autonomic nerves control blood flow, sweating, and skin moisture. Autonomic neuropathy is caused by a malfunction of those nerves. When this happens, you lose the ability to perspire or create the normal oils that protect and keep the skin moist. The result is dry skin that peels or develops deep cracks (fissures) that can be painful.

These cracks are mostly on the surface of the skin. They may appear to be deeper because the skin on either side of the crack thickens and makes them look deep. They are commonly found on the bottom of your foot where the toes bend or on the back of your heels. The danger associated with fissures is that they offer a "portal of entry" for bacteria, yeast, mold or fungus that can lead to an infection. And, as a person with diabetes, when you have an infection, it is much more difficult to treat, and is likely to take more time to heal.

SKIN PROBLEMS MAY REQUIRE A FOOT EXAM

Most people don't know the difference between dry skin and infected or diseased skin. If you have tried to treat your dry skin yourself and it doesn't go away, or if you see it spreading to other parts of the body or to other people, it is likely that you make have a skin infection. Skin problems may be viral (such as warts), fungal (such as tinea infection or athlete's foot), bacterial (such as cellulitis or infection), or cancerous (such as melanoma).

Dry, itching skin can also be caused by a failure of the veins in your legs to function correctly; this results in fluid collecting in the legs. This problem can lead to "venous stasis dermatitis," where the skin of the legs can become discolored, dry and itchy. Scratching this type of dry skin can cause a venous leg ulcer. In advanced cases, rust to orange-brown discoloration can be seen in the skin. This change

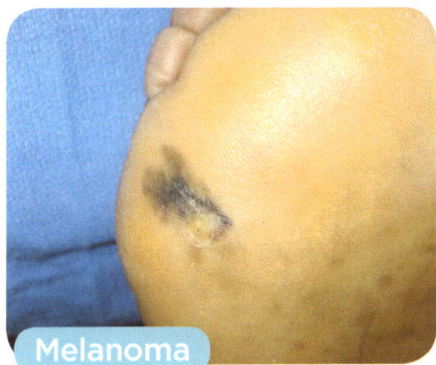

Melanoma

in the pigmentation of the skin is the result of iron from the pigment in the red cells depositing in the skin and oxidizing, much like an iron "I" beam that is exposed to the weather. An ulcer should be seen as a wildly waving red flag that gets your attention, particularly if you have diabetes.

TREATING DRY SKIN

If you have dry skin, use an emollient lotion containing urea. Urea has the unique ability to moisturize dry skin by drawing moisture into the cell structure in the top layer of the skin. It is available in several strengths and is one of the best products for this condition. If you can't reach your feet, recruit a family member or friend to help you apply lotion.

Hydrating the skin is one behavior that actually helps to prevent ulcers and amputations.

ADVANCED SKIN PRODUCTS

Skin can be nourished from the outside in with advanced nutritional products. There are many worthwhile skin care products containing specific, specially-treated amino acids, antioxidants, MSM (methylsulfonylmethane), a naturally occurring anti-inflammatory agent, and vitamin co-factors which can nourish and strengthen the skin, providing an insurance policy against skin breakdown, trauma, such as skin tears and wounds. These products not only improve the skin's appearance and texture, but also help build collagen and develop the skin's resistance to damage, which is very important for people with diabetes. Advanced skin care products additionally provide high-tech protection due to their ingredients, such as quality silicones, like dimethicone, zinc oxide, calamine and surfactant-free phospholipids — cleansers that clean with derivatives of vegetable oil instead of harmful, drying detergents or soaps. In recent research, advanced skin products have additionally been shown to substantially decrease the incidence of pressure ulcers and skin tears and to drive down associated costs with these troublesome wounds.

SKIN SUBSTITUTES

Treatment Options for Healing Diabetic Foot Ulcers

Doctors who treat wounds are using bioengineered dressings (Apligraf™, Dermagraft™) for a variety of wound needs, including delivering growth factors and specialized cells. These products produce an immediate cover and support healing. A unique topical medication,

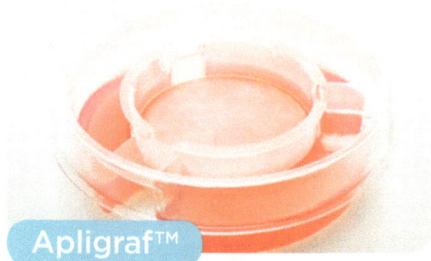
Apligraf™

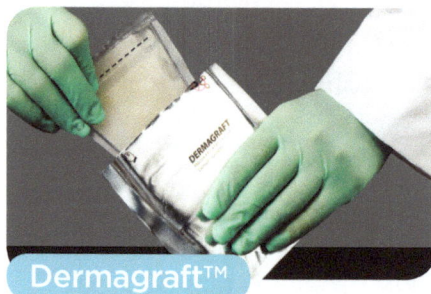
Dermagraft™

Regranex™ Gel has been successfully used to heal diabetic foot ulcers.

"Regranex® Gel contains becaplermin, a recombinant human platelet-derived growth factor for topical administration." Recent research has revealed "an increased rate of mortality secondary to malignancy was observed in patients treated with 3 or more tubes of Regranex® Gel."

Platelet-derived growth factors can be used to produce a wound gel that is actually created from the individual's own blood to stimulate healing. This therapy is being used more not only for healing diabetic foot and venous leg ulcers, but also for treating sports injuries.

Using stem cells to heal wounds that previously resisted healing is an exciting and growing area of science.

CHAPTER 9
NAILS

> From an evolution standpoint, toenails make complete sense. They are a leftover from when feet were used more like hands, serving a similar function to fingernails, helping to open vital food objects, strip bark to build structures, protection, etc.
>
> — Unknown

Toenail issues often cause pain or functional disabilities for people with diabetes. Nails are frequently difficult to care for at home and people with diabetes often cut themselves while trimming their nails. Toenail problems can be a "trigger" that can lead to more serious foot disorders, such as foot ulcers, infections, and amputations.

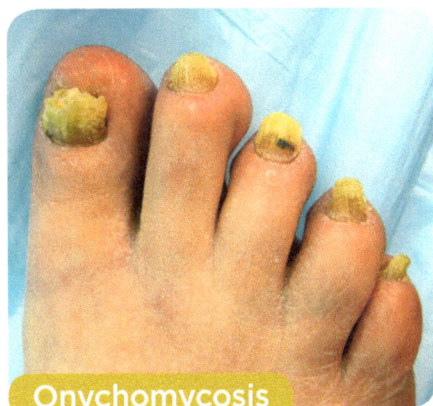

Onychomycosis

TOP TOENAIL TIPS

Do's

1. Trim your nails using nail files with coarser sandpaper (such as used for artificial fingernails). Filing is less risky than cutting.

2. Trim your nails with the contour of the toe, being sure all sharp edges are cut or filed smoothly.

3. Keep your toenail length even with the end of the toe.

4. Seek medical attention right away for any injury that does not heal promptly. If you have nerve damage or poor circulation, and you cut yourself, contact your provider immediately.

Don'ts

1. Don't cut your own toenails if you can't do it safely.

2. Don't use pocketknives, sewing scissors, or your teeth to cut/bite your nails. Don't pick at your toenails with your fingers.

3. Don't attempt to cut or trim thick toenails; your foot care specialist has special tools and is trained to trim thick nails.

4. Don't assume that if you don't feel pain in your foot caused by a toenail that you don't have a foot problem, or even an injury.

SHOULD YOU CUT YOUR OWN TOENAILS?

Here's a quick guide to help you decide whether or not you should cut your own toenails. If you have any doubt, don't do it. You can ask a friend or family member for help, or go to a podiatrist. If you have diabetes and nerve damage or poor circulation, Medicare or private insurance may cover the cost of having your toenails cut.

YES, IF …

1. Your vision is good.

2. You can reach your feet.

3. You are careful.

4. You have good quality nail clipper.

NO, IF …

1. Your vision is impaired.

2. You are overweight, have arthritis or have other problems that make it difficult for you to reach your feet.

3. You have thick or deformed nails.

4. You have nerve damage or poor circulation, causing numbness in your feet.

Clippers

If you decide you can cut your nails, use good quality nail clippers. They should be easy to hold in your hand, clean, dry and sharp, though it is not necessary that they be sterile. If the blade is dull, you will have to use more pressure to cut your toenails, and you are more likely to cause an injury. Either have the blade sharpened or replace your clippers with a new sharp one.

Injuries

There are no guarantees about safe cutting of toenails. Even though you are careful, you may accidentally cut yourself. If you

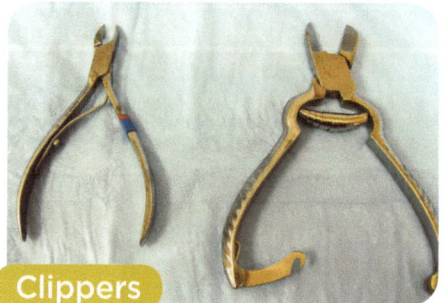

Clippers

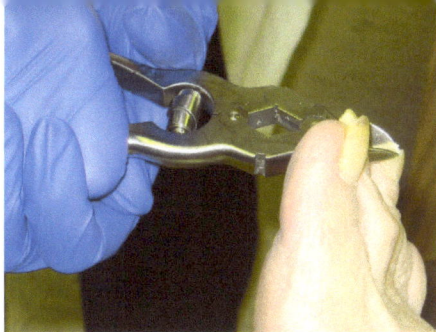

do injure yourself, follow these steps immediately:

1. Wash the injured area with soap and water.

2. Pat dry.

3. Apply an antiseptic cream and put on a loose bandage that does not cut off your circulation.

4. Change the bandage and inspect the injured area daily.

5. Ask for help if you can't see or care for the injury.

6. Report the injury to your health care provider immediately if the area turns red, swells, feels warm, or is not healing. Over-the-counter antibiotics are not strong enough to cure infection in the feet of people with diabetes.

Pedicures

While some nail boutiques are extremely conscientious about sterilization of instruments and sanitary practices, unfortunately, many are not. If you have diabetes, a pedicure can unnecessarily expose you to risk. First, it disturbs the skin and cuticle, which serves as a protective seal around your nails. Second, technicians use instruments that are able to draw blood and that carry the danger of transferring bacterial organisms. Sharp, cutting instruments like nail clippers, may or may not be sterile or used by a trained technician.

Naturally, cosmetology is focused on aesthetics. It is the exception rather than the rule to find a technician who has even the most rudimentary knowledge about diabetes, skin and nail infections.

The most important issue, however, is that you can't go to a salon for a pedicure and expect to have a professional available to diagnose your foot and nail problems, recognize your risk factors, educate you about preventing foot diseases, and provide you with legitimate treatment. For more information on pedicures read, "Death by Pedicure" by Dr. Robert Spaulding. (www.justfortoenails.com.)

Podiatrists advise people with diabetes to avoid pedicures in a non-professional environment because they know the special training needed to perform diabetic foot care, which includes taking care of your toenails.

NAIL DEFORMITIES

Perhaps the most common of all foot problems involves the toenails, and there are several types of problems that can affect the nails. The nails may be invaded by dermatophytes, mold, yeast, fungus, or even by bacteria. Ingrown toenails and thickened and deformed nails are also very common.

Damaged Nails: Totally Dystrophic Nail Syndrome

If you hit your nail against an object, like a doorframe or chair leg, or drop something on it, your nail will suffer what is called "blunt force trauma." When this occurs on the matrix, the area that the nail grows from may be damaged. If so, it will produce a nail deformity called totally dystrophic nail syndrome.

Sometimes, this is mistakenly diagnosed as a nail fungus. Medications will not cure this syndrome. Treatment may include debriding (cleaning) or reducing the thickness of the nail. In some cases, people prefer to have the nail permanently removed.

Ingrown Toenails

An ingrown toenail is a common problem for people in general, and can be more dangerous for people with diabetes. It is a painful condition that occurs when a piece of nail gets imbedded in the soft tissue adjacent to the nail.

At the base of the nail, under the skin, there is a specialized tissue called "the matrix" from which the nail grows. Think of the matrix as an envelope. The cells are on top and underneath, and the nail comes out from in between the two surfaces of the matrix. If you get an ingrown toenail, it's probably caused by the way your nail is trimmed. You may have left a little piece near the edge or trimmed the nail too far back along the nail border. As the nail grows out, it eventually becomes imbedded in the soft tissue next to the nail. However, some people have inherited curved nail borders, and are always fighting ingrown toenail problems.

An ingrown toenail is a mechanical problem that must be locally treated. If you have diabetes, do not attempt to solve this problem on your own. You may make the problem worse, or break the skin and develop an infection. Even if you are taking antibiotics, the problem is likely to recur once the antibiotics

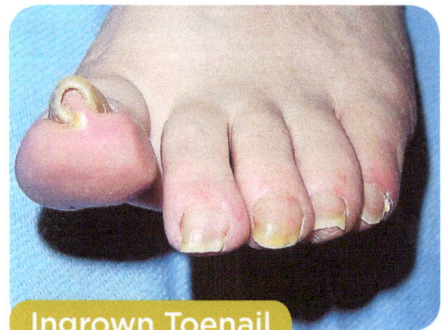
Ingrown Toenail

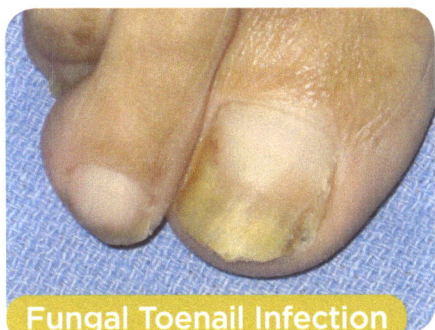

Fungal Toenail Infection

have been stopped. To make this problem go away, a portion of the nail needs to be trimmed to stop it's pressing against the skin. This may or may not solve the problem permanently. If the problem recurs, your foot care specialist can permanently remove a portion of the side of the nail. This painless procedure is done under local anesthesia in the doctor's office.

You will need to wear a surgical shoe after the procedure so the freshly operated foot doesn't go into a closed and perhaps unclean shoe, and there will be some local after care until the site heals.

Nail Infections

Fungus, mold and yeast infections of the nails — live infections that are contagious to others — are a common problem. In fact, 60% of the world's population suffers from these infections. People with diabetes are affected even more frequently. A "mycotic" infection will cause the nail to thicken and change color from its normal pink to yellow, green, or brown. A deformed and thickened toenail can scrape the adjacent toe and cause an ulcer. Toenail deformities can also cause an abscess to develop under the toenail as a result of pressure from the shoe against a thickened nail. (An abscess is a collection of pus that accumulates in a cavity of tissue.)

If you have lost protective sensation for pain, have poor vision, or don't inspect your feet, you may not be aware of this problem until there is pus or blood on your socks, and by then, it is usually too late. Once you have a soft tissue infection that goes unattended, it may turn into a bone infection. This type of infection may be difficult to resolve without prolonged therapy of intravenous or oral antibiotics and surgery to remove any infected bone.

Fungal infections of the toenails not only impact the condition of the nail, they can also cause psychological issues, physical pain, and limit a person's ability to walk and enjoy life. If you are a person with diabetes who has lost protective sensation for pain in

Keep your toenail length even with the end of the toe.

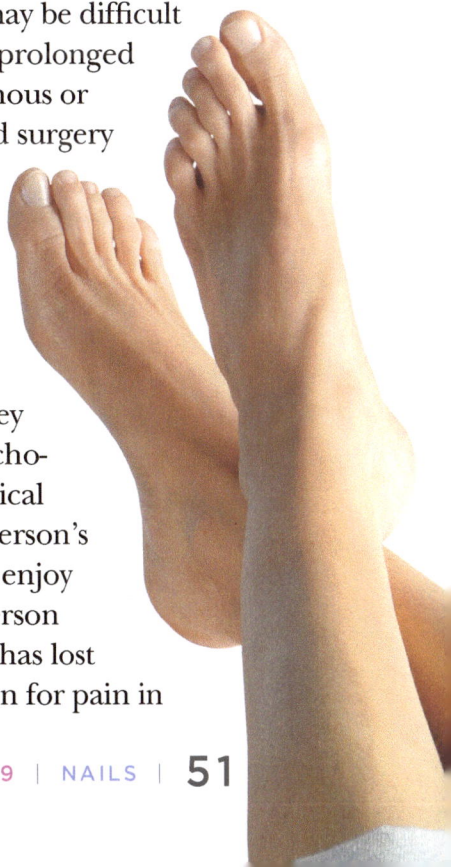

✓

SELF CARE TIPS IF YOU LOSE A TOENAIL

Keep area clean

Don't go barefoot

Wear shoes with extra room for your toes

your foot—peripheral sensory neuropathy —and you also have a toenail deformity, you really should have professional foot care. Your podiatrist can clean (debride) and trim the nail to prevent abscesses and lacerations. (cuts)

Bacteria do not usually affect toenails, but mold, yeast, and fungus (also known as dermatophytes), seem to thrive on skin and nails. A nail infected with a dermatophyte infection is called onychomycosis, which means nail (onycho) fungal infection (mycosis).

The two most common fungal organisms that cause onychomycosis are in the Trichophyton family of organisms; T-Rubum and T-Mentagrophytes. If the skin on your feet is red, swollen, and itchy, chances are that you have an infection caused by a dermatophyte.

Fortunately, there are now several safe and effective oral (can be taken by mouth) antifungal medications, Lamisil™ and Sporanox™, available to

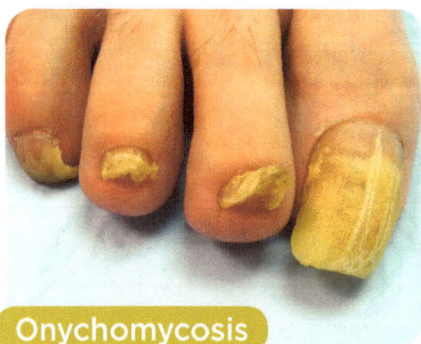

Onychomycosis

treat these infections. However, if you have had hepatitis or have liver disease (diagnosed by elevated liver function tests), you should not use these medications. Some people have reported using tea tree oil or Vicks Vapo Rub™ on their nails to resolve dermatophyte infections, but there is no scientific evidence to prove these treatments work.

TOENAIL INJURY

A toenail that has suffered direct blunt trauma may develop a blue tingled color under the nail bed. This is called a subungual hematoma (sub = below, ungual = nail, hematoma = collection of blood). This type of injury can be very painful. When the collection of blood under the nail is surgically drained, the discoloration will go away and the pain will be relieved. After a toenail injury, an infrequent complication can be that the nail falls off. Usually, the nail will grow back within 12-18 months; however, it may have a different shape. If you lose a toenail, here are a few tips in self care.

- Keep the area clean and dry.

- Protect yourself from further damage (don't go barefoot).

- Wear shoes that have plenty of room for your toes.

CHAPTER 10
COMMON FOOT PROBLEMS

> The foot is an engineering masterpiece and a work of art.
>
> — Michelangelo

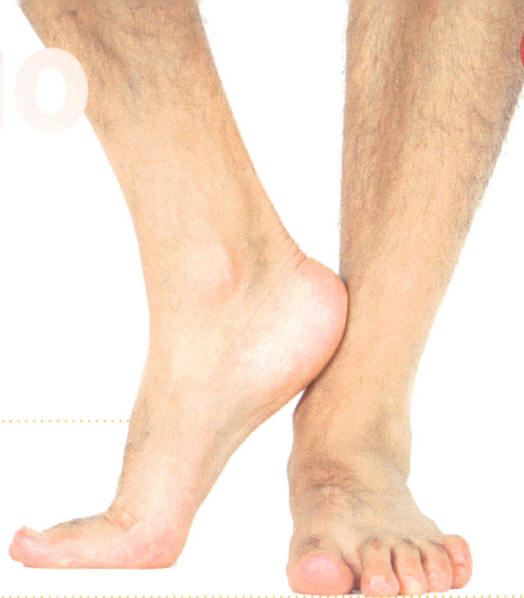

People with diabetes have many of the same foot problems as people without diabetes, such as corns, calluses, bunions and ingrown toenails. But, what appears to be an ordinary foot problem is more serious for you if you have diabetes and also have nerve damage or poor circulation.

YOU MAY HAVE A PROBLEM IF YOUR FOOT IS...

- Smelly: Foot odor can sometimes be a symptom of a serious problem that has not been detected, such as an infection or an ulcer.

- Red

- Warm

- Filled with pus

- Tender

- Painful

- Swollen

- In an abnormal position.

- Not able to have weight put on it.

TOP TIPS

Do's

- Try to determine what is causing the problem.

- Seek professional help.

Don'ts

- Don't use over-the-counter corn and callus removers, especially if you have nerve damage. They are made of harsh chemicals, usually acids, and should not be used by people with diabetes.

- Never try to remove a callus or corn by cutting or trimming it with a razor blade or other sharp cutting instrument.

CUTS, SCRATCHES

Here are the steps to follow if you have cuts or scratches on your feet:

1. Promptly wash the area with warm water and mild soap.

2. Use a mild antiseptic, such as Bactine.™

3. Cover the area with a dry, sterile dressing. Avoid adhesive tape or dressings that may pull off skin when removed, such as adhesive bandages.

4. Rest with your foot elevated.

5. Call your health care provider if the area involved does not improve within 24 hours.

ATHLETE'S FOOT

If you have itchy, burning, red, soggy, flaky, cracking skin, or dry scales between your toes on the soles or sides of your feet, you most likely have athlete's foot or tinea pedis. To confirm athlete's foot, your health care provider needs to look at skin scrapings under a microscope or send a tissue sample to the laboratory for analysis. However, it is often treated without this testing.

Here are the steps to follow if you have athlete's foot:

1. Practice better hygiene. Wash your feet help to prevent infections. Rinse and dry well, especially between your toes.

2. Check with your health care provider about the appropriate antifungal powder, spray or cream to use. A doctor can prescribe a stronger antifungal cream or pills.

3. When using a cream, apply a thin layer, at least twice a day (morning and night) for at least 4 weeks.

4. Do not use bleach on your feet, it can burn your skin and does not kill the fungus.

5. If you experience redness, swelling, a locally warm area on your foot, or pus, see your health care provider right away.

6. You can lace a little lamb's wool between your toes to keep the area dry (do not use cotton balls or tissues; they increase the pressure).

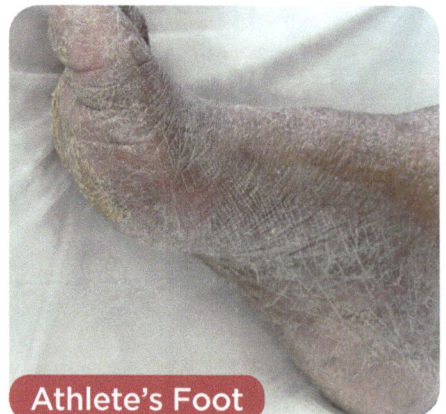

Athlete's Foot

To avoid getting Athlete's Foot, here are some prevention tips:

- Keep your feet clean and dry; avoid excessive perspiration and dark, warm, moist environments.

- Wear socks with fibers that carry the moisture away from the skin.

- Wear a clean pair of socks every day.

- If your feet get wet, change your socks more often.

- Use talcum or foot powder on your feet.

- Wear shoes with uppers made of leather or fabric that allows air to pass through.

- Allow shoes to dry between wearing.

- Wear swim sneakers at the beach or pool.

BLISTERS: A SIGN OF FRICTION

When there is an abnormal rubbing or friction against your foot from an improperly fitted shoe or other foot gear, the skin layers separate and your body responds by creating a fluid filled "pillow," called a blister. Here are the steps to follow if you have a blister:

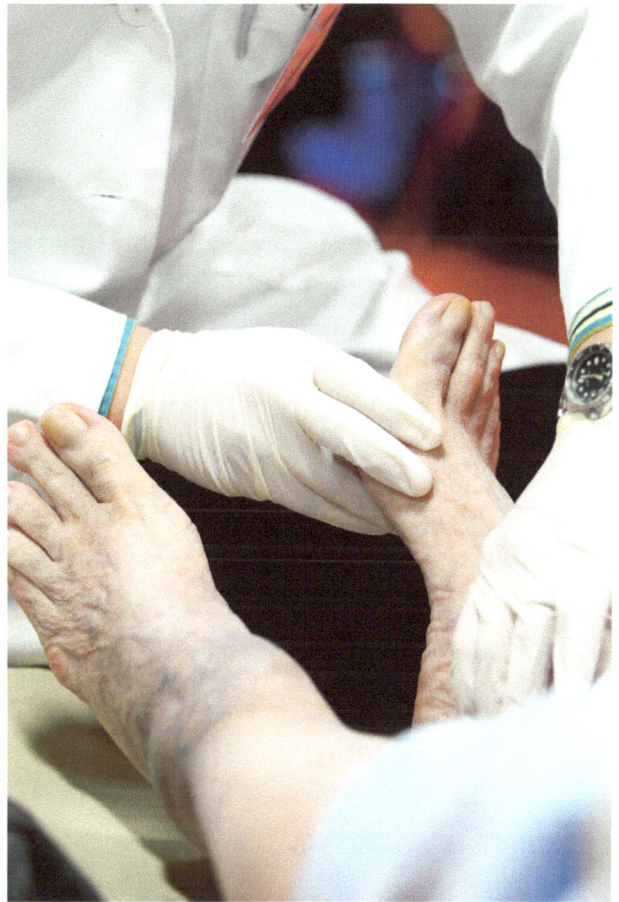

1. Stop wearing the shoe that might be causing it. You might need extra padding or different socks to avoid the friction; however, you might need to discard the shoes.

2. Wash the area with warm water and mild soap.

3. Rinse well and dry well, especially between your toes.

4. Cover the blister with a dry bandage (do not break the blister).

5. If it breaks, leave the loose skin as a covering over the wound until it heals.

6. Do not apply any ointments or medication to the blister.

7. Inspect the blister daily.

8. If the blister is red, tender, swollen, very warm, or filled with fluid after the first day, you may be getting an infection. See your health care provider to get antibiotics. Over-the-counter creams are usually not strong enough.

9. If the wound is deep, gets larger, or doesn't heal in a few days, see your foot care professional right away.

10. If the blister is not caused by friction, you might have a condition called diabetic bullae (fluid-filled blister), which is fairly rare. However, you should follow the same care routine.

Blisters in the diabetic foot usually change into ulcers, which can become the trigger for infection and amputation.

STUBBED TOE

Here are the steps to follow if you have a stubbed toe:

1. Put ice on the injury

2. Elevate it higher than your heart to relieve swelling and pain

3. See a healthcare provider if your toe is in an abnormal position, you have continued pain or swelling, or you can't put weight on your foot

4. If you have nerve damage or peripheral vascular disease, and you cannot feel pain, look carefully at your toe and your foot and check it with your hands. If you see blood under the toenail, or if the injury looks severe, see your health care provider for an X-ray to evaluate for a fracture.

PUNCTURE WOUNDS
Stepping on a Nail or Foreign Object

A puncture wound is dangerous; over and above the puncture wound itself, a piece of the sole or insole from your shoe may have been forcibly pushed into your foot.

Here are the steps to follow if you have a puncture wound:

1. If you have nerve damage or poor circulation, see your health care provider immediately.

2. Wash the area with warm water and mild soap.

3. Dry well.

4. Cover the wound with a dry bandage.

5. Don't apply any ointment.

✓

YOU MAY HAVE A PROBLEM IF YOUR FOOT IS

Smelly

Red

Warm

Filled with pus

Tender

Painful

Swollen

Abnormally positioned

Not able to bear weight

6. Change your bandage daily.

7. Inspect the wound daily for redness, swelling, pus, or drainage. If you notice any issues or experience higher blood sugar than normal, see your health care provider.

8. Have a tetanus booster every 10 years; it is safe to have one if you have just been injured.

9. An X-ray should be taken to see if there is any foreign material embedded within your foot. Caution – non-metallic materials such as shoe sole or insole materials may not be revealed in an X-ray. If there is persistent infection, surgery may be necessary to open the wound, cleanse it and remove any foreign material that may be inside your foot.

DIGITAL (TOE) DEFORMITIES:
Hammertoes, Claw Toes, Mallet Toes or Overlapping Toes

These deformities usually mean that you have had a change in the position of your foot bones or a tightening of the tendons in your toe or toes. Toe deformities can cause corns, hard tissue growths on the top or on the tip or between curving toes that can be the triggers for ulcers.

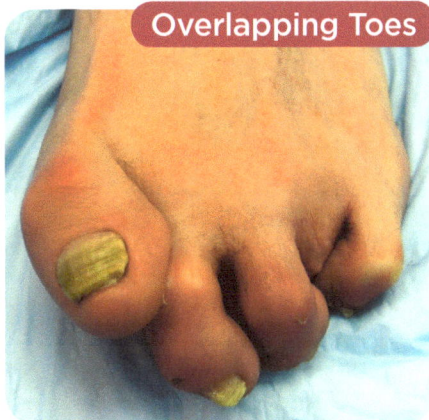
Overlapping Toes

Here are the steps to follow if you have these toe problems:

1. Throw out the shoes that are causing the problem.

2. Purchase shoes with a soft, rounded, and deeper toe box and a soft insole under the toes.

3. Pad the toe. Make sure the corn pad does not have chemicals.

4. Inspect your feet daily.

5. See your health care provider if the corn needs trimming or becomes irritated and changing shoes doesn't help; you may need orthotics or surgery to accommodate or correct the problem.

CORNS & CALLUSES

Keratosis is the medical term for these soft tissue lesions of the foot. They are formed by nature to protect your feet when there is abnormal pressure against

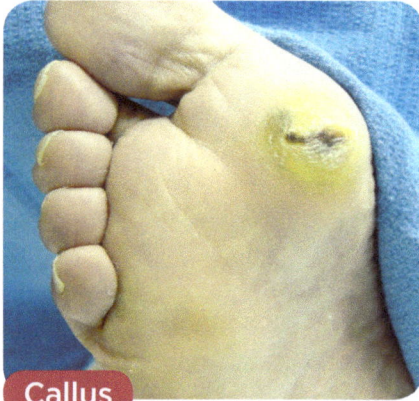
Callus

a bony structure. A soft corn, called a heloma molle, is located between your toes and is kept soft by the moisture between the toes. The bones in adjacent toes rubbing against each other cause it. A hard corn, called a heloma durum, is typically located on the top or distal tip of a toe. Calluses are typically located under the metatarsal heads on the bottom of the foot and are often mistaken as warts.

A callus can be thick and hard and can make it feel like you have a rock in your shoe if you can feel it. The biggest problem with a callus is that the tissue beneath it can become damaged or abscessed; that is how most foot ulcers on the bottom of your foot begin.

Here are the steps to follow if you have a callus:

1. Try to decrease or offload the high pressure on that spot; you may need to change shoes.

2. Wear shoes with soft insoles and cushioned outer soles.

3. Moisturize the skin to keep it soft.

4. Use an emery board, a callus file or a pumice stone to gently sand down the callus. Buff a little every day after a bath or shower when the skin is still damp. Do not scrub too hard.

5. See a foot health care provider to determine what is causing the callus.
   - Corns and calluses can be trimmed by your podiatrist for foot comfort and to prevent ulcers.
   - If the callus is very thick, you may need to get orthotics to offload the pressure from the callous site.
   - You may benefit from surgery to correct these deformities permanently.

Here are the steps to follow if you have soft corns between your toes:

1. Change to a shoe that is wider in the front.

2. Loosely lace lamb's wool or some special toe separator pads made of soft foam rubber or silicone through the toes. Do not use cotton balls or tissues.

3. Inspect your feet daily.

4. See your foot health care provider if the corns needs

trimming or becomes irritated. If the corns persist, you may benefit from surgery to correct the problem causing the corn.

PLUGGED-UP SWEAT GLANDS

Porokeratosis is a common skin lesion that is usually found on the non-weight bearing surfaces of the bottom of the foot. It appears as a small seed-like skin lesion or a miniature callus. It is often misdiagnosed as a wart.

WARTS

Plantar warts are caused by the papilloma virus, which can get under skin on the bottom of the feet. It may be difficult to tell the difference between a plantar wart and a callus. If a wart is improperly removed, it can leave a painful scar on the bottom of your foot, which may affect your walking.

Here are the steps to follow if you have a wart:

1. Leave it alone if it is not painful, but monitor it.

2. Your healthcare provider may trim, pad, or remove it with a chemical acid, liquid nitrogen, surgery or a laser. The problem with these treatments is that if ever one cell is left, another whole lesion can come back, and usually with a vengeance. The best way to treat warts is by using a laser beam that destroys all the wart cells.

3. People with diabetes should NOT use over-the-counter medications to self-treat warts.

BUNIONS

If you have an unsightly bump in the joint behind your big toe, you likely have a bunion. A bunion is the result of the big toe joint being out of alignment. The first metatarsal bone begins to move toward the opposite foot and the great toe moves in the opposite direction, toward the fifth or small toe of the same foot. At times, the second toe may overlap the great toe. Normally, the great toe joint functions as a freely-moving hinge. It's not supposed to rotate or move crossways; only up and down. Because of the deformity, the head of the first metatarsal can rub against the

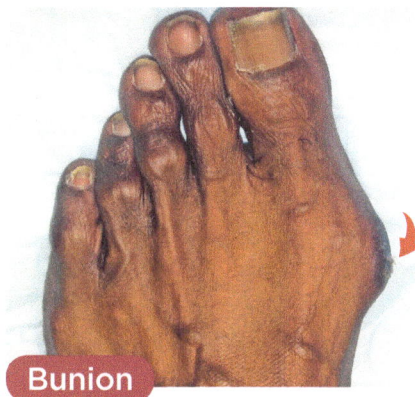

Bunion

BONE SPURS

Bone spurs can occur on any bone in your foot; however, they are usually seen on the bones of the toes. These sharp points of bone can cause small, painful skin growths between the toes called heloma molle, a keratosis also called a soft corn. Surgical smoothing of the bone spur will eliminate the painful keratosis.

HEEL PAIN

If you are overweight or have a job that involves standing — such as a beautician, food service worker, or cashier—or if your work involves walking or standing on hard concrete floors, you may be subject to heel pain.

While there are a variety of causes of heel pain, the most common reason for heel pain is plantar fasciitis, an inflammatory condition of the supporting structure called the plantar fascia. The plantar fascia runs from the toes to the heel and acts as a shock absorber. If you have had plantar fasciitis for some time, the chronic internal bleeding associated with it can cause calcification of the fascia where it attaches to the heel bone, resulting in a heel spur. Treatment options include rest, cortisone injection(s), orthotics, physical therapy, stretching exercises, anti-inflammatory medications,

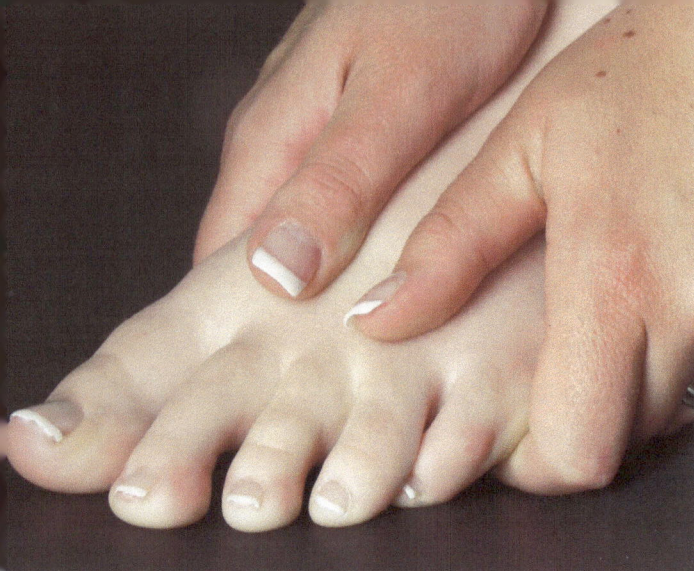

shoe and cause a blister. This bone deformity is dangerous if you have diabetes because you can develop an abscess or ulcer, which can become infected and lead to a bone infection. A tailor's bunion is similar to a bunion of the great toe joint, except that it occurs at the fifth toe joint. It too, is the result of a misalignment of the bones of the joint. A bunion can be caused by:

- Faulty biomechanical function.
- Uneven weight distribution during walking.
- Abnormal stresses in your joints.
- Wearing shoes with pointed toes.

If you have a bunion, see your foot healthcare provider to discuss special shoes, orthotics, padding, or surgery to remove the bump, re-align the joint and control the mechanical problem that caused it with biomechanical orthotics.

and application of ice or surgery. See your foot health specialist to find out your specific problem and treatment alternatives.

CHARCOT FOOT

Charcot foot is a severe foot deformity of the mid-foot; the scientific name is neurogenic arthropathy. It is a result of altered nerve function that occurs when a person has chronically elevated blood sugars. It is very difficult to heal; in some cases, it can take more than a year. Charcot foot is seen in people with diabetes and is the result of increased blood flow to the mid-foot that robs the bones of their mineral content. Hundreds of micro fractures occur and this leaves you prone to develop an ulcer in the mid arch area of your foot. If you have Charcot foot, the mid-part of your foot literally collapses because the bones give out. It's rarely painful, but it does cause the foot to become unstable.

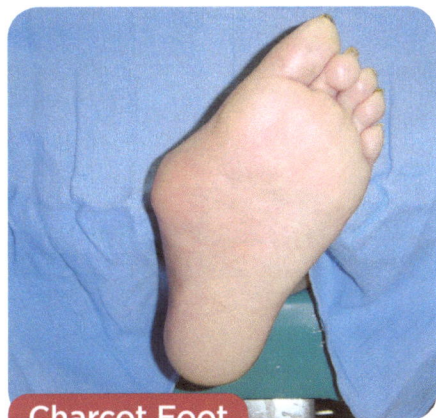
Charcot Foot

If you notice changes in the structure of the middle of your foot, see your healthcare provider. It can be difficult to diagnose, because it may appear as a bone infection. Lab testing, X-rays, as well as bone and soft tissue scans may help in determining if there is joint inflammation, fractures, dislocations, or an infection of the soft tissues or bone. Charcot foot can be treated using a cast-like device called a cam walker, or a total contact cast or it may be repaired with reconstructive surgery.

NEUROMA, FOOT TUMORS and CYSTS

A non-cancerous (benign) tumor of nerve tissue, or a neuroma, is a common problem seen in the feet of women more than men. This condition occurs where the nerve passes between the bones in the front of the foot just behind the toes and gets pinched. When there is pressure against the nerve (such as when the bones are pinching), the nerve sheath begins to swell to protect itself, and can become a space-occupying mass that can be extremely painful. It can be difficult to know the source of this foot pain, especially in a situation where there are other related problems that affect the foot, including diabetic sensory neuropathy, tarsal tunnel syndrome (a compression of the nerve behind the ankle), and lumbar radiculopathy (a nerve condition that causes pain to radiate from the back that may reach down to the foot). In the person with diabetes, pain in the foot that is commonly diagnosed as diabetic peripheral sensory neuropathy, may in fact be a pinched nerve in the foot ankle or back. Since there are a number of clinical problems that can cause foot pain, it is possible that a person with diabetes can have both problems at the same time, so the diagnosis of foot pain in the person with diabetes can be challenging. Your foot care specialist can examine you and help to determine the reason for your foot pain.

Tumors of the foot do occur, but luckily, the majority of them are benign. The most common noncancerous tumors of the foot are lipoma (a tumor of fatty tissue), fibroma, (a tumor of fibrous connective tissue), and neuroma. Cancerous tumors found on the foot include: Kaposi's sarcoma, and malignant melanoma, and are fairly rare.

Cysts, like ganglions, are fluid-filled soft tissue masses that usually originate from the joint capsule or tendon sheath. They usually contain a viscous fluid are easily felt (palpable) and are easily treated.

TUMORS OF THE FOOT DO OCCUR, BUT LUCKILY, THE MAJORITY OF THEM ARE BENIGN.

Another area for tissue problems is the bottom of your foot and the chambers of fat pads located under both the front of the foot and the heel. You can have tumors of the fat pad (lipoma), derangements of the fat pad, or you can lose the fat pad. This usually happens under the forefoot, which leaves the metatarsal heads unprotected and prone to ulcers. This is most commonly seen in people with rheumatoid arthritis. If you have a hard, round, raised skin structure on the bottom of your foot, called a nodule, it could be a rheumatoid nodule, a giant cell tumor of tendon sheath, or a fibroma, which is a benign tumor of connective tissue. Fibromas have a very high recurrence rate and should only be surgically removed with caution. Orthotics can help offload the pressure, which lessens any pain associated with these tumors.

PAIN

Pain, The Gift
Nobody Wants
— Dr. Paul Brand

I n 1993, Dr. Paul Brand wrote, *Pain, The Gift Nobody Wants.* In this book, he tells his life story and shares his discoveries about pain. He was the first physician to understand the "Gift of Pain" and learned the tragic results when people lose this "gift" while working with the patients with leprosy in India. Later in his life, while working in the United States, he was the first physician to understand and link the problems of sensory neuropathy that robs patients of the "gift of pain," that he learned about with patients with leprosy to patients with diabetes.

Pain is your body's burglar alarm. It lets you know when your body has been injured.

While the following explanation of how diabetes affects your foot was discussed earlier in the book, it bears repeating. Chronically elevated blood sugars cause your circulation and your nervous system to function poorly or improperly. The smallest arteries, called arterioles, become narrowed or even blocked when your blood sugars remain high. When this happens, the artery can't provide your nerves with fresh oxygenated blood and nutrients, so your nerves don't work as they should. Eventually, the nerves fail. For people with diabetes, this malfunction can result in the loss of vision, loss of kidney function and loss of protective sensation for pain to the feet, which is called diabetic sensory neuropathy (DSN). Without the ability to sense pain, your foot is vulnerable to mechanical, thermal, or chemical trauma. *(See Chapter12)* Although the initial damage may seem minor, these injuries are often the "triggers" that can start a process that causes soft tissue damage, leading to infection, ulceration, hospitalization, and amputation.

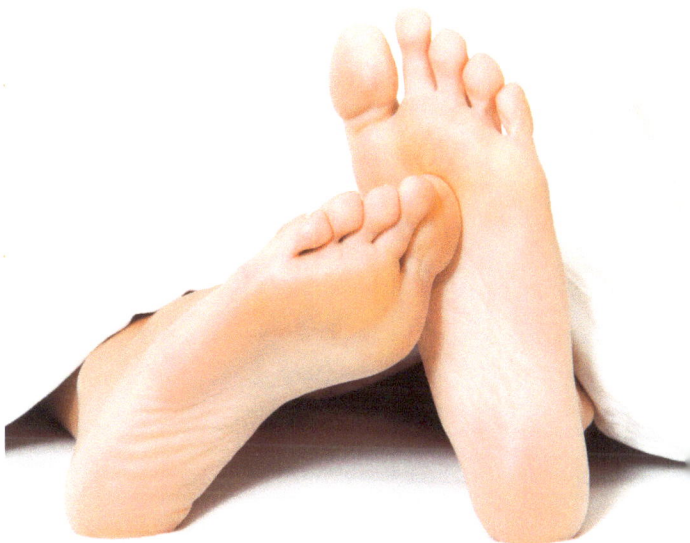

So, if you have been injured — even though you might not feel pain — and your foot has

In this chapter

PAYING ATTENTION TO PAIN

TREATING PAIN

HELPFUL PRODUCTS

Stop wearing the shoe that might be causing a blister.

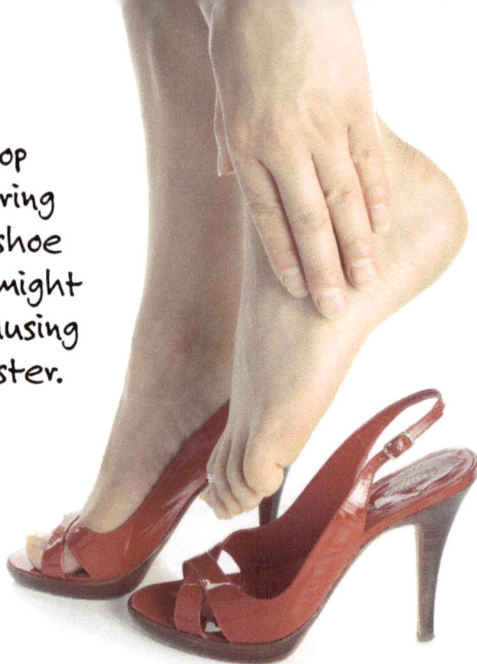

TOP TIPS

Don't
Never use the following therapies without recommendations from your physician:
• ice pack
• hot foot soak
• ice or gel packs that you can either freeze or heat in the microwave

an opening in the skin, becomes red, swollen, or has a local increase in temperature, you MUST see your foot care specialist right away to prevent complications.

Diabetic sensory neuropathy robs a person of the ability to feel the "gift of pain;" however, not all people with diabetes lose the ability to feel pain. This condition tends to happen after blood sugars have been elevated or uncontrolled over a period of time. So, the decisions you make today concerning maintaining blood sugars will have consequences later in your life. If for no other reason, this is why it is critically important for people with diabetes to keep their blood sugars in the normal range.

Still, pain is a symptom common to many foot problems.

DO PAY ATTENTION TO PAIN

Many people choose not to see a doctor when they have foot problems. Having pain is a red flag that should not be ignored. If you have any of the following foot health issues, see a foot care specialist immediately.

1 **Heel pain** is usually caused by soft tissue inflammation, but can also be the result of a broken bone, a tight Achilles tendon, a pinched nerve, arthritis, or other problems.

2 **Ankle sprains** require prompt medical attention. If they are not treated, you increase your risk of repeated sprains and of developing chronic ankle instability and pain.

3 **Big toe stiffness** and pain usually develop over time as the cartilage in the big toe joint wears down and eventually leads to arthritis. The sooner a doctor diagnoses it, the easier it is to treat.

4. **Achilles tendonitis** causes pain and tenderness at the back of the foot or heel. This is usually the result of a sudden increase in physical activity. The risk of an Achilles tendon rupture can be reduced by promptly treating the symptoms.

5. **Ingrown toenails** can pierce the skin, allowing bacteria to enter your body. A foot care specialist can perform a quick procedure under local anesthesia that will stop the pain and permanently cure an ingrown toenail.

6. **Pinched Nerve, Neuritis, or Neuroma.** People with diabetes tend to have more nerve problems. These problems can affect the front of the foot, as well as the heel and the ankle. The most common nerve problem in people with diabetes is a burning, shooting, tingling, or numbing feeling in the area of the toes and just behind the toes on the bottom of the foot. In some people, the entire foot might feel numb. Problems of the nerves are commonly misdiagnosed as diabetic sensory neuropathy. *(See Chapter 12)* While DSN can cause foot pain, pain could also be the result of other problems. One is radiculopathy, which is foot pain that is caused by a back problem. Another is a pinched nerve behind the ankle, called tarsal tunnel syndrome. If you have a pinched nerve in your foot or ankle, a steroid injection may give you instant relief from the pain.

Testing is available to identify each of the possible reasons for your pain, so there is no need to suffer pain when it can be diagnosed and treated.

If you have foot pain, get a foot exam to determine the nature of your pain and get it treated.

TREATING PAIN

The following are some over-the-counter and prescription products that may help resolve your pain:

Analgesics are orally administered pain relievers, such as acetaminophen, which relieve pain without relieving inflammation. Pain relievers should only be used after a legitimate evaluation has been made, rather than as a method of self-treatment.

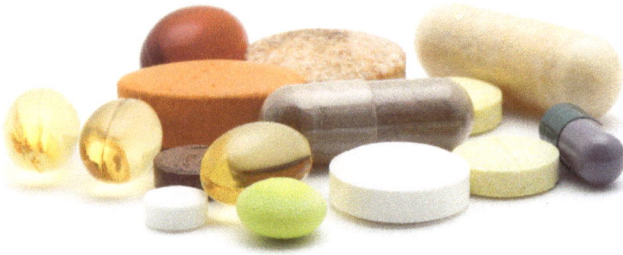

Topical analgesics are lotions, creams, or gels applied to the skin where they penetrate to relieve mild foot pain.

- Some topical preparations containing menthol, eucalyptus oil, or turpentine oil reduce pain by distracting the nerves with a different type of sensation. Neurogen,™ an over-the-counter topical medication, has successfully been used for pain management. Another type of topical analgesic delivers salicylates (the same ingredient as in aspirin) through the skin.
- Topical Lidocaine Gel 5% is another medication that can be applied to the skin that numbs it and relieves pain.
- Another topical medication, Capsaicin,™ counters a chemical known as substance P, which is a neurotransmitter that transmits pain signals to the brain. Capsaicin™ is derived from a natural ingredient found in cayenne pepper. For that reason, it may burn or sting when first used. Be sure to use gloves when applying Capsaicin™ to the body. Getting this product in your eyes would be severely painful.

Non-steroidal anti-inflammatory drugs (NSAIDs) include aspirin, ibuprofen, Motrin™ Advil™, and naproxen (Aleve™).

Opioid analgesic drugs contain opioids such as codeine, hydrocodone, or morphine and provide stronger pain relief because they block certain chemical pathways that send pain signals through the central nervous system. These drugs may only be prescribed by your doctor. Nerve pain medications are prescribed for pain caused by nerve damage that does not respond well to opioids. A nerve block injection can numb a particular nerve to prevent pain signals from reaching your brain.

Corticosteroids are synthetic forms of naturally occurring hormones produced by the adrenal glands. These may be given topically, in pill form, or by injections to decrease inflammation and relieve pain. Topical corticosteroids, applied directly to the skin, are useful only in treating rashes. Pills and injections are used for treating nerve entrapments* and musculo-skeletal and arthritic pain, but these drugs must be used wisely. They do incredible things, but they can also cause atrophy (weakness due to decrease in muscle mass) of the skin, increase blood sugar, elevate blood pressure, and negatively affect soft tissue.

Oral medications, such as Gabapentin, Neurontin™, Lyrica™, or Cymbalta™, can help to relieve that pain associated with diabetic sensory neuropathy. Alpha Lipoic Acid in combination with Vitamins C and E can also help to reduce pain.

Non-narcotic pain management The Regenesis Biomedical Provat Pain Management System relieves pain without drugs.

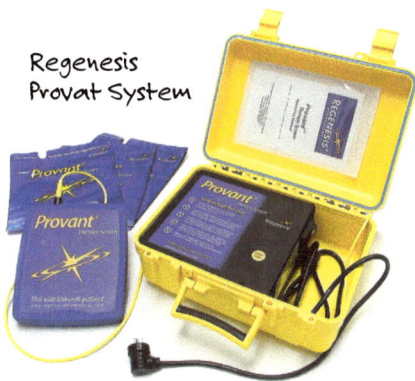

TESTING IS AVAILABLE TO IDENTIFY EACH OF THE POSSIBLE REASONS FOR YOUR PAIN, SO THERE IS NO NEED TO SUFFER PAIN WHEN IT CAN BE DIAGNOSED AND TREATED.

FACTS

Regenesis
Provat System

Nerve entrapment: repeated, long-term harmful pressure on a nerve, usually near a joint that is subject to inflammation or swelling

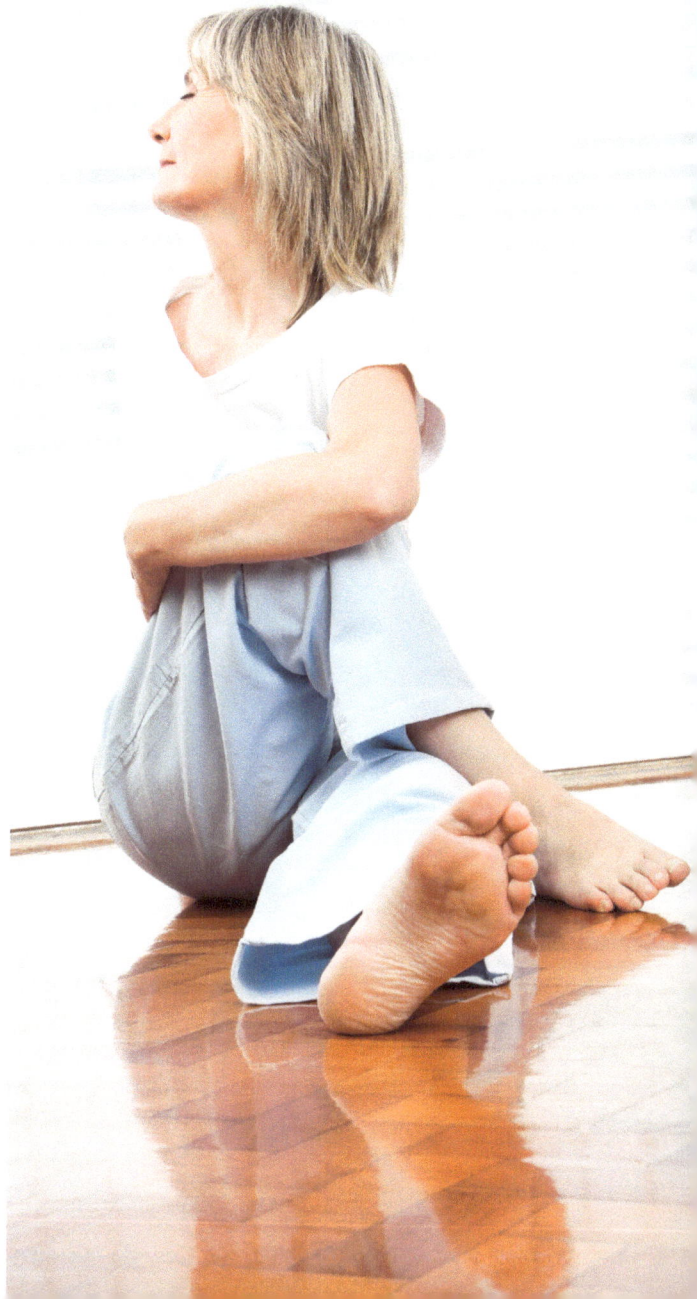

EASY-TO-APPLY PRODUCTS AVOID DISCOMFORT

When you have a wound that requires a dressing, the last thing you need is one that causes pain every time it needs to be changed. There are pain-reducing dressings available that combine silicones for gentle no-stick, pain-free dressing changes. These include super-absorbent foam materials.

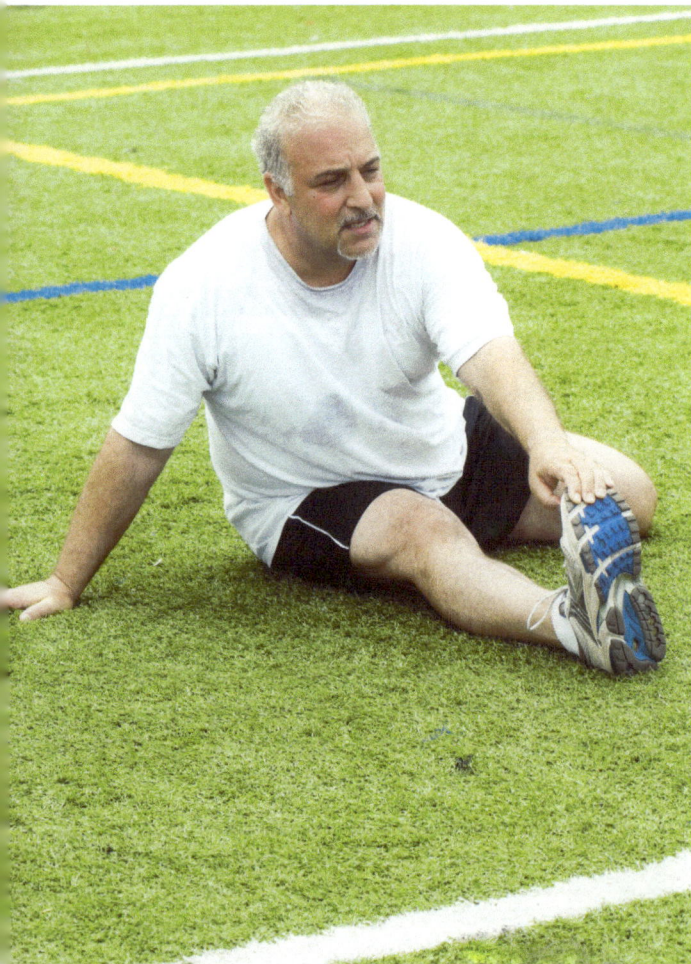

PAIN-FREE PRODUCTS INCLUDE ALCOHOL-FREE, NON-STINGING PREP WIPES AND SPRAYS TO PROTECT FRAGILE, WOUNDED SKIN FROM DAMAGE AND FROM ADHESIVE STRIPPING.

Other pain-free products include alcohol-free, non-stinging prep wipes and sprays to protect fragile, wounded skin from damage and from adhesive stripping. These easy-to-apply co-polymers provide protection for the vulnerable skin without the pain and stinging sensation that alcohol-based ones might create.

If you have foot pain, get a foot exam to determine the nature of your pain and get it treated.

CHAPTER 12
NERVE DAMAGE
OR
NEUROPATHY

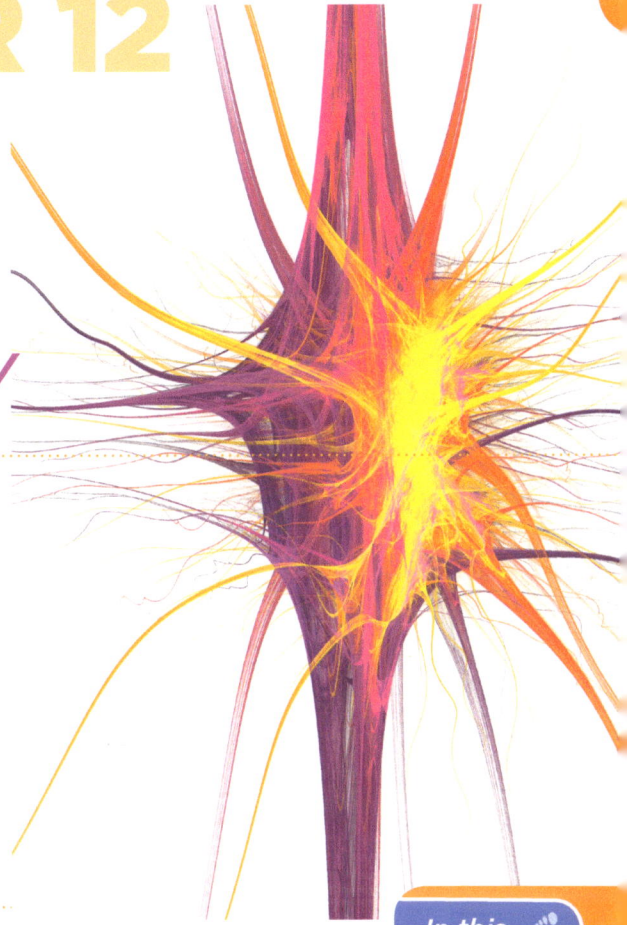

Although peripheral diabetic neuropathy most commonly affects feet, it can also impact the legs, arms, and hands. Nerve damage first appearing as discomfort, tingling, and extreme sensitivity to touch may graduate to severe pain, followed by numbness.

Seventy-five percent of all people with diabetes have nerve damage, also known as "neuropathy." Once you have nerve damage, there is no going back. Read about what can happen if you have nerve damage, and resolve to prevent these problems by keeping your blood sugar levels close to normal.

Sustained or chronic high blood sugar levels most often cause nerve damage in people with diabetes. However, exposure to heavy metals, such as lead or mercury; chemicals; pesticides; herbicides; radiation; chemotherapy, excessive alcohol intake, vitamin deficiencies and antibiotics can also cause it.

PERIPHERAL NEUROPATHY

If your nerves are not transmitting neurological impulses normally, you may have peripheral neuropathy. Peripheral means "at the edges or away from the center;" neuropathy refers to changes to the nervous system.

Every person who has peripheral neuropathy is unique, with different symptoms and complaints. Some people get a sensation similar to when you hit the "funny bone" in your elbow. Others describe PN as feeling like they're walking on pins and needles, nails or glass, or like lightning bolts are shooting through their feet. Some describe it as feeling like they are standing on a balled up sock or on wood. Worse yet, some people have no feeling at all in their feet. They liken it to when your foot "falls asleep;" that is, they can't even feel the floor while standing.

SYMPTOMS OF NERVE DAMAGE

If you have one or more of the following symptoms, you may have Peripheral Neuropathy:

- Muscle weakness
- Cramps
- Numbness
- Tingling
- Pins and needles
- Burning sensation
- Night time foot or leg pain
- Fainting, vomiting
- Changes in bowel, bladder, sexual functioning

The medical terms you may hear your doctor use for these symptoms include:

- **Parasthesia:** the sensation of a little lightning bolt shooting through your foot.
- **Hyperesthesia:** the foot is extremely sensitive to touch;

sometimes even just getting under the bedcovers can cause extreme pain.

- **Hypoesthesia:** a decreased sensitivity to light touch and vibratory sensation, so that you can't even feel the fibers of a brush or a vibrating tuning fork applied to the foot or ankle.

TYPES OF NEUROPATHY IN DIABETES

In people with diabetes, chronically elevated blood sugars start a chain reaction that results in either the loss of, or severe changes to, nerve functions. People with diabetes are typically affected with one of three different types of neuropathy caused by these nerve function changes. Each one has different signs and symptoms.

MOTOR NEUROPATHY
Damage to the nerves of your muscles.

As a person with diabetes, you have been told how important it is to keep your blood glucose levels in a normal range. One important reason is that chronically elevated blood glucose levels can damage your nervous system. Subtle changes in your nerve function may lead to your losing muscle mass and power in your foot muscles. This is known as "motor neuropathy."

Motor neuropathy occurs when the nerves that supply the foot muscles, the Lumbracles and Interossei muscles that control fine movements of the toes, are damaged. Weak muscles can result in a change to the shape of your foot, especially the toes. Motor neuropathy will cause your toes to shift into abnormal positions, resulting in a variety of digital (toe) deformities.

Hammertoe is the term used to describe a deformity of the smaller or lesser toes where the toe becomes shorter or tighter (contracted) at the point of attachment or proximal joint. The result is that ligaments and tendons have tightened causing the toe's joints to change position. Thus, the top of the toe tends to rub against the shoe.

Mallet toe describes a toe where the joint at the end of the toe cannot straighten, causing the tip of the toe to rub against the shoe.

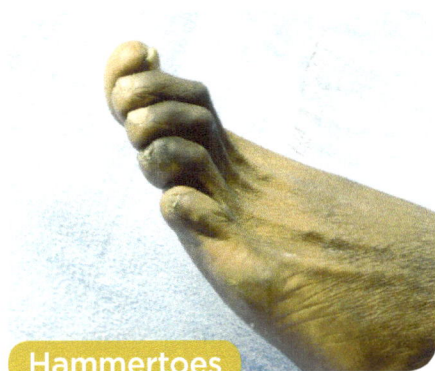

Hammertoes

Claw toes occur when ligaments have tightened, causing all of the toe's joints to contract. The bony prominences in the toes caused by these deformities can become triggers for mechanical injuries; for example, corns may develop on the toes. Sometimes, the normal fat pad on the bottom of the foot shifts and can't protect the bones in the front of the foot. These changes may create new pressure points and change the way you walk (your gait) and you will develop a callus. Unfortunately, soft tissue lesions, such as corns and calluses, can be the triggers for soft tissue infections.

Using magnetic resonance imaging (MRI) technology, scientists have been able to see the smallest muscles in the foot. They found that people with diabetic motor neuropathy have muscles that are smaller when compared to people without motor neuropathy. These findings also suggest that changes in the muscles occur early, often before other recognizable other changes to the foot associated with neuropathy are noted.

AUTONOMIC NEUROPATHY
Damage to nerves that control automatic body functions.
If the nerves that aren't functioning in your body are those

SEVENTY-FIVE PERCENT OF ALL PEOPLE WITH DIABETES HAVE NERVE DAMAGE, ALSO KNOWN AS "NEUROPATHY."

SYMPTOMS
OF NERVE
DAMAGE

Muscle
weakness

Cramps

Numbness

Tingling

Pins and
needles

Burning
sensation

Night time
foot or
leg pain

Fainting,
vomiting

Changes in
bowel,
bladder,
sexual
functioning

responsible for controlling automatic body activities, you may have autonomic neuropathy. This might affect your blood flow, your digestion, as well as your major body systems: your heart, stomach, sexual organs, eyes, and bladder.

The malfunction of these nerves impacts the sweat or oil glands in the skin of your legs and feet. When this happens, you can lose the ability to perspire or create the normal oils that protect and keep your skin moist. The result is that you will have dry skin that peels or develops deep openings or cracks (fissures) that can be painful. While these cracks are on the surface of the skin, there is a thickening of the skin on either side of the crack that makes them look deeper. They are commonly found on the bottom of your foot where the toes bend or flex and on the back of the heels.

The gravest danger of these cracks or fissures is that they offer a "portal of entry" for bacteria, yeast, mold or fungus that

Fissure Heels

can lead to an infection. And, once you get an infection, it is much more difficult to treat. If you have autonomic neuropathy and are experiencing dry skin on your feet, use a moisturizing cream or lotion daily to keep the skin moist.

SENSORY NEUROPATHY
Damage to the nerves that control your ability to sense pain resulting in Loss of Protective Sensation for Pain (LOPS).

No one likes to feel pain. But not being able to feel pain may be even worse. By far the most dangerous complication of chronically elevated blood sugars is this loss of protective sensation for pain known as Diabetic Sensory Neuropathy or DSN.

Pain is your body's burglar alarm. It alerts you to intruders such as injuries. It has existed in humans from the beginning of time; and, as unpleasant as it may be, humans would not survive without it. Without the ability to feel pain, our bodies are vulnerable to a variety of injuries, or traumas. As a matter of fact, after pulse, respiration, blood pressure, and temperature, pain is considered to be the fifth vital sign. Without the ability to feel pain, you are vulnerable to being injured without realizing it.

The ability to feel pain is controlled by your sensory

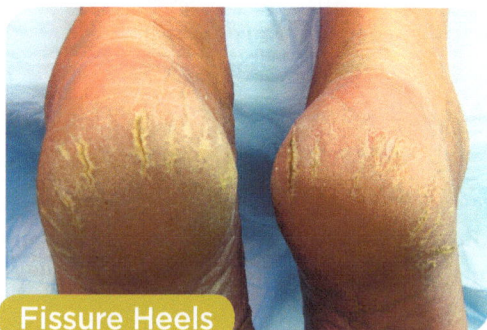

nerves. They give you information about your environment, and that includes a sense of where your joints are positioned and input from mechanical and thermal receptors that can generate impulses that you recognize as pain.

Sensory neuropathy, therefore, is the most dangerous of the three types of neuropathies, because people affected by sensory neuropathy can get injured without knowing it. They have lost the ability to feel pain, or what is called a loss of protective sensation for pain (LOPS), and are vulnerable to painless trauma of mechanical, thermal or chemical origin. (See below for details)

If you have diabetes and have the type of nerve damage that impacts your ability to sense pain, you may not notice if you have a foot injury, a sore, or even a high pressure area. If you then continue to walk on your feet despite this problem, a simple issue can become a dangerous wound or ulcer. Peripheral diabetic sensory neuropathy is generally the greatest risk factor and often the root cause for foot ulcers in people with diabetes. Just because you do not feel pain in your feet, doesn't mean you should ignore a foot injury. A hole in the foot is not harmless, even if it is painless.

Not being able to feel pain with your feet goes beyond ulceration. It may also impact your ability to feel temperature differences, so you may not realize it when your feet are in water that is too hot or too close to a an artificial heat source. Lack of feeling in your feet also impacts your sense of balance, which may cause you to have more falls.

You may not realize how the ability to sense feeling in your feet communicates to you exactly where you are positioned in your three-dimensional world, until you lose that feeling.

PAINLESS TRAUMA

Here are three ways you could painlessly traumatize your feet. Each type of trauma is a trigger that can start the process of injury that can result in infection, ulceration, hospitalization and amputation. You should learn about them so you can avoid these potential hazards to your foot health.

Mechanical Injury

Mechanical injuries are those that are caused by a physical process. They may result from minor trauma, such as bumping your foot into a door frame; stepping on a sharp object, like a nail; or rubbing against a foreign object, like a stone, inside

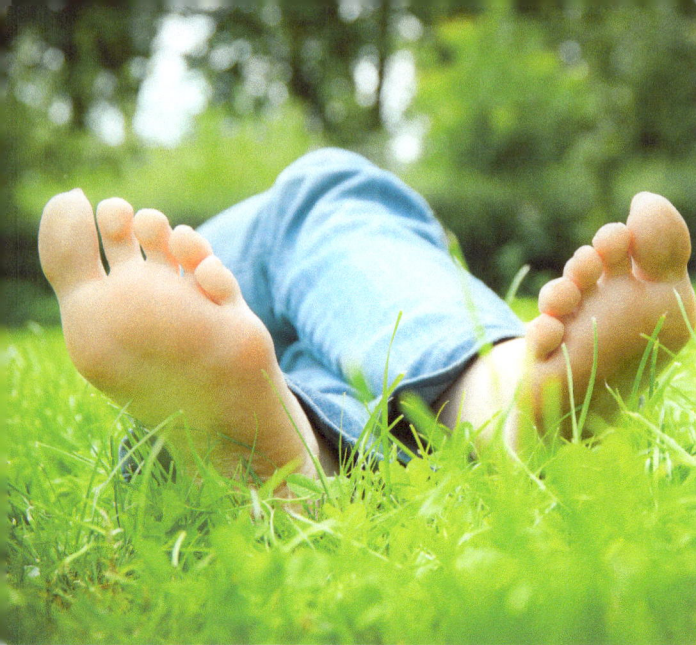

sory neuropathy and have lost the ability to sense pain in your feet, it is very important that you are aware of the potential for injury when you are trying to warm your cold feet. These injuries can result from trying to warm feet using a heating pad, a hot water bottle, an open fire, a radiator, a hot brick or hot water in a foot-fixer bath.

Chemical Injury

Over-the-counter products for treating foot problems usually contain salicylic acid, which destroys tissue painlessly. Salicylic acid is also found in medicated corn pads and in topical wart, ingrown toenail, and callus removers. But the acid eats everything it touches — both the affected tissues and the healthy skin. Avoid using over-the-counter products for your foot care and seek professional care from your foot specialist.

the shoe, or an improperly-fitted shoe. They can also be caused by deformities of the bones, soft tissue, or nails interacting with footgear. For example, a toenail thickened by fungal infection can rub against another toe and scrape it or rub against the shoe and cause a blister or an abscess. If you also have poor circulation, this type of injury can start the sequence of events that ultimately could lead to an amputation.

That is why it important to get properly fitted footwear, to check inside your footwear for any objects, and to check your feet daily.

Thermal Injury

Injuries relating to temperature are called thermal trauma. They may result from overexposure to heat or to cold. Most foot related thermal traumas are burns caused by an artificial heat source. If you have diabetic sen-

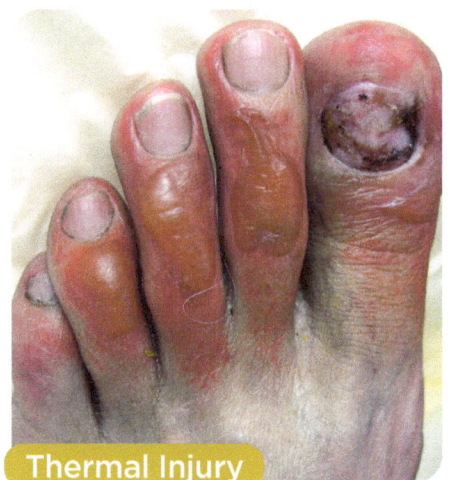

Thermal Injury

DIAGNOSIS

There is no cure for diabetic neuropathy, but awareness and care can prevent complications which could become severe enough to warrant amputation. After taking your medical history, here are some tests your doctor may perform to determine if you have nerve damage:

1. Tests for
   - range of motion
   - muscle power
   - skin evaluation
   - vascular evaluation
   - neurological response
   One of the first predictors of neuropathy in people with diabetes is the loss of deep tendon reflexes, which are the patellar (knee) and achilles (ankle) reflexes. You've probably had this test during check-ups—your doctor taps your knee and ankle tendons with the neurological hammer and your reflexes cause your leg or ankle to jump.

2. Examine your foot by touching (palpating).

3. Test for feeling on the bottom of your foot (loss or protective sensation for pain) with one of the following tests. If you have feeling, that means that your protective sensation for pain is intact. If you don't feel it, you have lost protective sensation for pain, so your foot is considered "insensate."

   - A monofilament-testing device (MTD) (plastic wire) is the gold standard (the most accepted medical practice worldwide) for detecting diabetic sensory neuropathy. The MTD tests your ability to feel a sensation on the bottom of your foot from the device that is pre-calibrated and standardized. The MTD is a reliable, fast, non-invasive, and painless test for diagnosing peripheral sensory neuropathy and LOPS.
   - An electronic tuning fork or bioestheometer is used to determine your ability to sense vibration.

4. The IPN (Indicator Plaster Neuropad) is a simple high-sensitivity device that can be used for diagnosing autonomic neuropathy. The IPN can be performed either in the office or by the individual or caregiver at home. It takes about 10 minutes.

TREATING PERIPHERAL NEUROPATHY

Your health care professional may recommend one of the following medical treatments for peripheral neuropathy. However, your

60-70% OF THOSE WITH DIABETES WILL DEVELOP PERIPHERAL NEUROPATHY, OR LOSE PROTECTIVE SENSATION FOR PAIN IN THEIR FEET.

best bet is PREVENTION: keep your blood sugar levels in the normal range and you most likely won't have to worry about nerve damage.

- Medications such as Neurontin™ (also known as Gabapentin) Lyrica™ or Cymbalta™.

- Vitamin therapy including Vitamins C, D, E and B complex.

- Drugs including narcotics; non-steroidal antiinflammatory drugs called NSAIDS, and tricyclic antidepressants, such as Amitriptyline™.

- Psychological counseling and emotional support for those who feel overwhelmed can be helpful.

Medical research has determined that low levels of vitamins B12, B6, and B1 can affect DPN. The best way to know if your neuropathy may have a component of vitamin deficiency is a simple fasting blood test. B Vitamins can be taken in pill form, patches, and nasal sprays. Vitamin B1 or Thiamine should be taken as the lipid soluble form of thiamine called benfotiamine. Dr. Richard Mann, CEO of Realm Laboratories, a manufacturer of a benfotiamine product called NeuRemedy, reports that this product is "a medical food that nourishes dysfunctional nerves allowing them to conduct impulses more normally. The specialized formulation in NeuRemedy contains benfotiamine. Benfotiamine has been used since the early 1960's to successfully help tens of thousands of patients suffering from peripheral neuropathy in Asia and Europe. It has been extensively studied in the scientific literature and has been shown to be safe and effective."

Damage to the nerves caused by chronically elevated blood sugars is the main reason for so much suffering and disability in the lives of people with diabetes. It is directly related to the increase in the cost of medical care. Your medical team can help you, but there are some things that only you can do, such as keeping you blood sugars under control. You CAN reduce your risk of developing the worst complications of diabetes and live a full and long life if you take an active role in keeping your blood sugars under control.

CHAPTER 13

WOUNDS

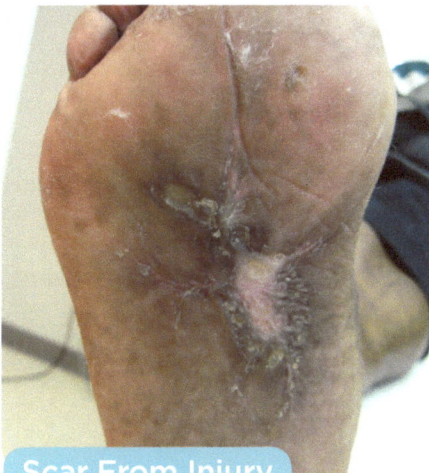

It's important to see
how we can advance in
healing wounds.

— Ricardo Lagos

If you have diabetes, you have a greater risk for complications from wounds. Because diabetes decreases your blood flow and alters the function of your immune system, your injuries are slower to heal than in someone who does not have the disease. If you also have peripheral sensory neuropathy; that is, you have lost protective sensation for pain in your feet, you won't necessarily notice an injury right away.

So, there's no such thing as a "minor" wound to the foot when you have diabetes; even a small

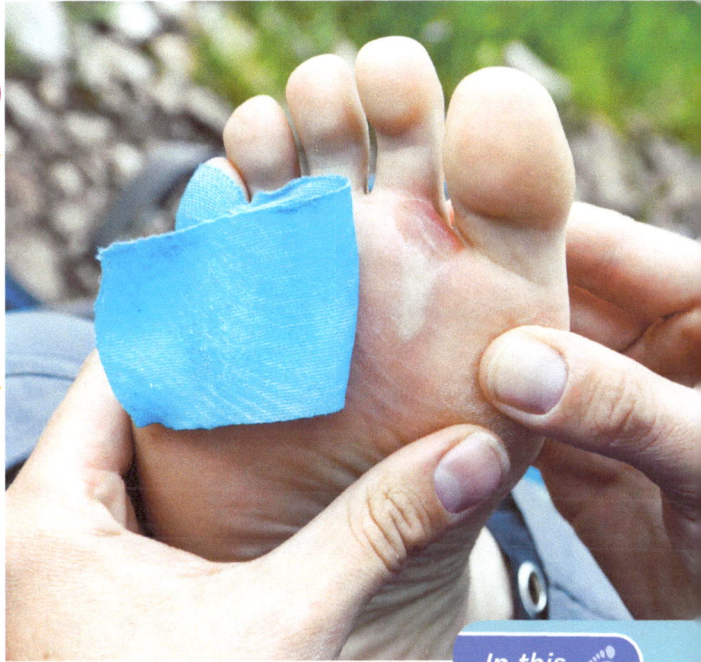

Scar From Injury

foot sore can turn into an ulcer that, if not properly treated, can lead to amputation.

When you are initially wounded and immediately treated, the wound may be called "acute," meaning that you have only had it for a short time and it is likely to heal quickly. A wound that is not continuously progressing towards healing is called "chronic," meaning that you have had it for a long time, or it frequently occurs, or that it is slowly becoming a more serious problem. Any wound that doesn't heal in four weeks is cause for concern, as it may result in a worse outcome, including amputation.

Unfortunately, foot ulcers in people with diabetes often become chronic.

In this chapter

MEDICAL ATTENTION

GOALS OF TREATEMNT

SPECIALISTS

CARE PRODUCTS

WOUND HEALING SKIN SUPPLIMENTS

PLATELET RICH PLASMA

POST TREATMENT

If you have a wound, here are some prompt actions you should take:

- Cleanse the wound with warm, soapy water and dry well.

- Put an antibiotic cream on the wound immediately.

- Cover the wound with a light gauze and keep pressure off the area.

- Do not wear closed shoes.

- See your foot care specialist or a local wound center within seven days at most if the wound has not responded to treatment.

MEDICAL ATTENTION

Once you go in to see the doctor about your foot wound, he or she may do several things:

1. **Test that you have good blood circulation to the area.** This exam is called an ankle brachial index. The results will determine if you should see a vascular surgeon for further examination and treatment.

2. **Take an X-ray** to be sure there is not a bone infection present.

3. **Clean your foot sore,** a process which is known as "debridement." The doctor may also take tissue from the area and send it to a labora-tory for culture and sensitivity to check the type of bacteria that may be present and determine the appropriate antibiotic to use to help heal the wound promptly. Debridement may be done at frequent intervals.

4. **Offload your foot.** This means finding a way to take the pressure off the wounded area of the foot. Avoiding all mechanical stress may involve putting your foot in a total contact cast (TCC) or other casts or support boots, surgical shoes, half shoes, sandals, or felted foam dressings. All of these will require you to walk with crutches. Bed rest may also be suggested.

5. **Application of extra cellular matrix dressings** or skin grafts that bring the specialized cells necessary to heal the ulcer to the ulcer bed.

6. **Platelet Rich Plasma.** A treatment that uses your own specialized cells that are removed from your blood, concentrated and placed into a gel and applied directly to the ulcer.

7. **Dress the wound to prevent further trauma,** minimize the risk of infection, and optimize the wound environment.

GOALS OF WOUND TREATMENT

Improve function

Healing foot wounds can improve your foot's appearance and function, so that you may walk better with appropriate footwear and conduct your daily activities on your own.

Control infection

Your health care team will do everything it can to prevent your wound from becoming infected. Infected wounds may involve deeper soft tissues or bone, and ultimately threaten your limb and even your life.

Maintain health

Diabetic foot infections may increase your blood sugar levels and can impact your ability to walk, move and function normally, which is not good for controlling your blood sugar, your kidney and heart function, or your nutritional needs. Not being mobile puts you in worse condition both physically and mentally.

Prevent amputation

If your foot wound can be healed, your risk of requiring an amputation is decreased. An amputation puts you at higher risk for a second amputation and also puts your life at risk. It also takes a heavy physical, emotional and financial toll.

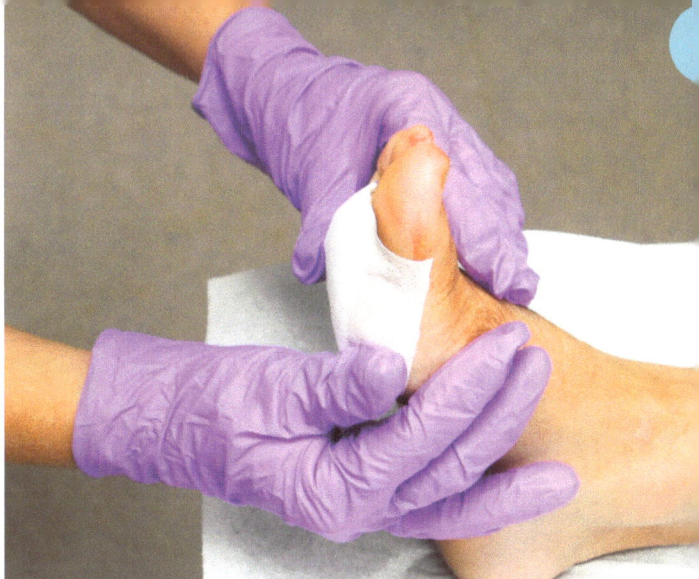

Reduce costs

An amputation is costly, and so is the follow-up treatment required after an amputation.

WOUND CARE SPECIALISTS

There are professionals who do specialize in wound care. You can find them through the American Academy of Wound Management (www.aawm.org). This free service helps people find certified wound specialists (CWS) in a specific geographical area. These professionals may be physicians, including podiatrists; nurses; or therapists. The Wound, Ostomy, and Continence Nurses Society (WOCN) has a similar consultant registry at www.wocn.org. The American Professional Wound Care Association (www.apwca. org) also has certified professionals in wound care including physicians, nurses, and therapists.

WOUND CARE PRODUCTS

Dressings

The primary function of a wound dressing is to promote a moist healing environment, which is necessary for wound healing. Dressings can range from plain gauze to sophisticated bioengineered tissue. Ask your doctor about the latest innovations in wound care dressings.

Never use a dressing that uses adhesive to secure it to your foot. Inevitably, during a dressing change, the adhesive will pull skin off of the wound, making matters worse. Non-adhesive dressings stick to themselves to secure wound dressings. While these dressings cost a bit more, the benefit in skin protection outweighs the risk of getting a wound complication.

There are many types of dressings for wound care that you and your caregiver can learn to use. Educational packaging usually contains easy-to-follow directions and information.

Antibiotic ointments & creams

Ointments keep a wound moist. Creams tend to dry up a moist wound. Most foot wounds are already moist; so, in the initial phase of healing, you want to dry them out. These wounds include ingrown toenails, abscesses, and cellulitis, a skin infection caused by bacteria. Use a cream-based antibiotic to help this type of wound dry out.

Any antibiotic cream or ointment you can buy over-the-counter is probably not going to be adequate to treat a serious infection; however, your doctor's prescription for appropriate antibiotics will likely be appropriate to treat your infection.

TREATMENT CHALLENGES

Some wounds have bacteria and dead tissue or even small parts of wound dressings in them and because they are not clean, they are a greater challenge to heal. This contamination of the wound is called "bioburden." Your doctor may consider using negative pressure wound therapy (NPWT) to clean the wound and accelerate wound healing. NPWT draws the wound edges together, provides a moist healing wound environment, promotes blood flow, removes wound debris and infectious materials, reduces swelling, and promotes tissue formation. You may also hear NPWT called topical negative pressure, sub-atmospheric pressure, sub-atmospheric pressure dressing, vacuum-sealing technique, or

GOALS OF WOUND TREATMENT

Improve function

Control infection

Maintain health

Prevent amputation

Reduce costs

sealed surface suctioning.

For healing of chronic, stubborn, or postoperative wounds, and to minimize the risk of infection, many experts recommend hyperbaric oxygen therapy (HBOT). This type of therapy can help heal wounds due to weakened immune systems and poor circulation. Healing tissue needs oxygen, and HBOT not only increases tissue oxygen levels, but it also improves the killing ability of white blood cells.

21st CENTURY ADVANCES IN WOUND-HEALING SKIN SUPPLEMENTS

Research has shown that most chronic wounds lack the necessary cells to heal the wound. In order to "jump start" the healing process of a wound or ulcer, skin substitutes containing the necessary cells to speed the process of wound healing can be used. The two products approved by the FDA for treatment of diabetic foot wounds are Apligraf™ and Dermagraft™. These specialized dressings contain the necessary cells to get the wounds back on track toward healing.

PLATELET-RICH PLASMA

The most difficult wounds to heal on the foot and leg are diabetic foot ulcers and venous leg ulcers relating to the veins

Wound care costs the US healthcare system more than $20 billion each year, including $4 billion spent on wound management products.

FACTS

or venous circulation that brings blood back to the heart. When conservative wound care and skin substitutes fail to heal the wounds, a treatment that uses the person's own blood usually works. The blood is spun in a centrifuge, and the serum with the platelets (small cells that start the wound healing process) is removed. Wound healing factors are added to the serum and it is then transformed into a gel that is applied to the person's wound. An astounding 93% of all wounds treated in this manner heal.

POST TREATMENT

After you've been treated for a wound, it is very important that you remain vigilant. Research indicates that among people who have had foot wounds, more than half develop another within two to five years. Regular visits to a podiatrist and wearing shoes with customized insoles designed to redistribute pressure along the foot can be helpful in preventing recurrence.

DIABETIC FOOT AND AMPUTATION STATISTICS

- Diabetes affects 27 million people in the US and more than 336 million people worldwide. [1]

- 60-70% of those with diabetes will develop peripheral neuropathy, or lose sensation in their feet. [2]

- Up to 25% of those with diabetes will develop a foot ulcer. [3]

- More than half of all foot ulcers (wounds) will become infected, requiring hospitalization and 1 in 5 will require an amputation. [4]

- Diabetes contributes to approximately 80% of the 120,000 nontraumatic amputations performed yearly in the United States. [5]

- Every 30 seconds, somewhere in the world, a limb is lost as a consequence of diabetes. [6]

- After a major amputation, 50% of patients will have their other limb amputated within 2 years. [7]

- The relative 5-year mortality rate after limb amputation is 68%. When compared with cancer — it is second only to lung cancer (86%). (Colorectal cancer 39%, Breast cancer 23%, Hodgkin's disease 18%, Prostate cancer 8%) [8]

- People with a history of a diabetic foot ulcer have a 40% greater 10 year mortality than people with diabetes alone. [9]

- Every 30 minutes, a limb is lost due to a landmine. Every 30 seconds, a limb is lost due to diabetes. [10]

- Having a wound immediately doubles ones chances of dying at 10 years compared with those without diabetes. [11]

1. Diabetesatlas.org/ American Diabetes Association, **2.** Dyck et al. Diabetic Neuropathy 1999, **3.** Singh, Armstrong, Lipsky. J Amer Med Assoc 2005, **4.** Lavery, Armstrong, et al. Diabetes Care 2006, **5.** Armstrong et al. Amer Fam Phys 1998, **6.** DFCon11, Bakker (after Boulton), DFCon. com Boulton, The Lancet (cover), Nov. 2005, **7.** Goldner. Diabetes 1960 Armstrong, et al, J Amer Podiatr Med Assn, 1997, **8.** Armstrong, et al, International Wound Journal, 2007 American Cancer Society; Facts & Figures 2000 Singh, Armstrong, Lipsky et al. J Amer Med Assoc 2005 Icks, et al, Diabetes Care, 2011, **9.** Iversen, et al, Diabetes Care 32:2193-2199, 2009, **10.** Bharara, Mills, Suresh, Armstrong, Int Wound J, 2009, **11.** Iversen, et al, Diabetes Care 32:2193-2199, 2009

CHAPTER 14
CIRCULATION

Dr. William Harvey authored On The Motion of the Heart and the Blood *in 1628 in Frankfort. This Englishman was the first person to offer a detailed description that accurately explained the body's circulation system.*

Poor circulation is 20 times more common in people with diabetes. Poor circulation is caused by plaque, made from fats such as cholesterol and triglycerides, which build up and harden in your arteries, and may block the blood supply to your foot. If you've had problems with your circulation in other parts of your body — if you've had a heart attack or a stroke, for example — you can expect to see the same circulatory problems affecting your feet and legs. The impact of diabetes on the circulatory system is cumulative. So, the decisions you make today concerning blood sugar control and practicing preventive behaviors have long-term consequences.

You are especially at risk of having circulation problems if your habits include smoking, eating sweet and fatty foods, and if you don't exercise. Those habits will result in high blood fat levels and poor blood sugar control.

In an active person, the movement of muscles will help blood and fluids circulate from the heart and back again. If you are not active, your heart may become too weak to pump blood around your body, Due to gravity, the fluid will collect in the lowest part of your body, and your feet and ankles will suffer.

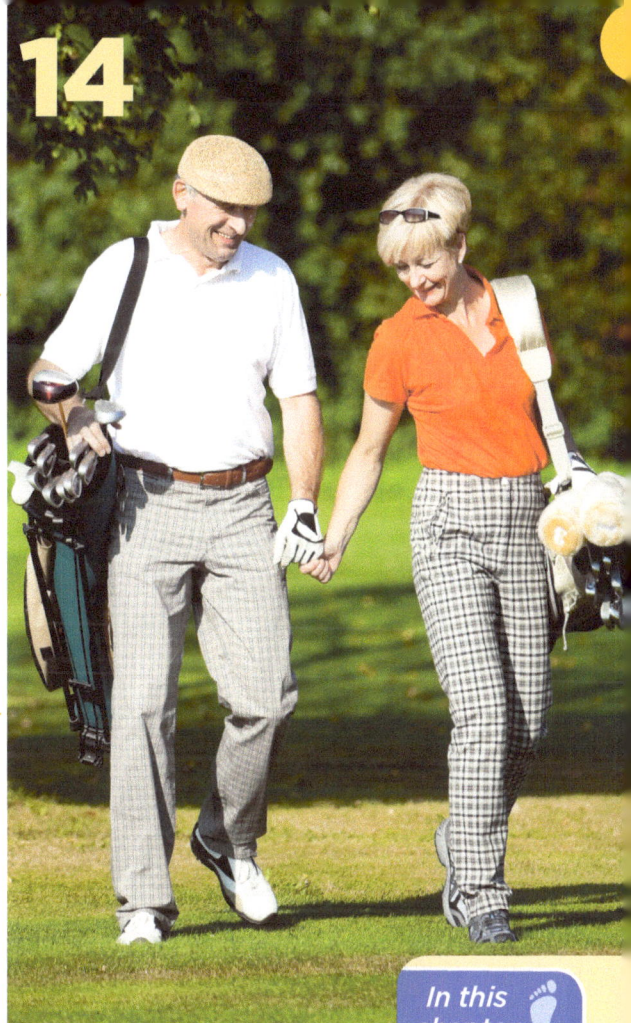

In this chapter

DO'S & DON'TS

SIGNS OF PROBLEMS

SKIN COLOR

COLD FEET

SWOLLEN FEET

DISEASES DIAGNOSIS

IMPACT ON FOOT WOUNDS

TREATMENT

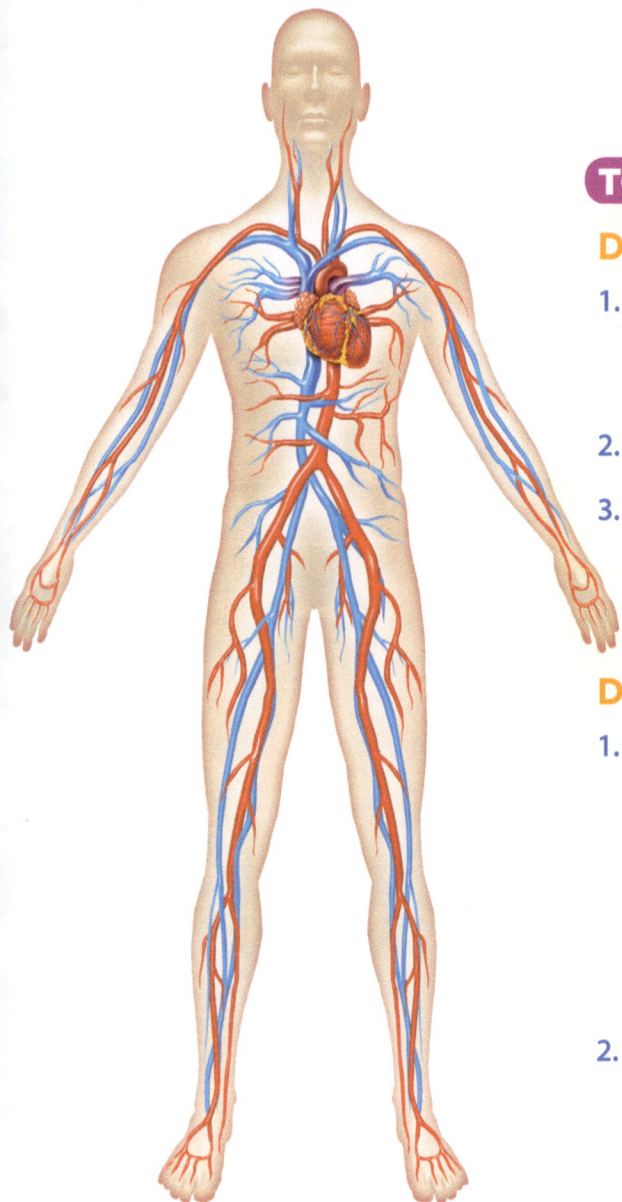

Do's

1. Stay active. Move your feet. The force of your contracting leg muscles helps blood and fluid return to the heart.

2. Put your feet up when you are sitting.

3. Wiggle your toes for five minutes, two or three times a day. Move your ankles up and down and in circles to improve blood flow in your feet and legs.

Don'ts

1. When sitting, do not cross your legs or ankles. If you must sit for a long period of time, use range of motion exercises to aid circulation. If you're on an airplane or in a car for a long period, get up or out and walk around every hour or two to help your circulation.

2. Do not wear any type of garter, girdle, or constricting garment that may impede circulation.

YOUR CIRCULATORY SYSTEM

The medical term for your circulatory system is the vascular system. It affects the function of every system and organ of your body. There are three parts to that system: the arterial, venous, and lymphatic systems.

The Arterial System carries blood from the heart through both large and small vessels to the organs and the extremities. The large vessels are found in the core of the body and extend out to the extremities; the small vessels are found within the organs and at the end in the extremities.

The Venous System returns the blood from the organs and

extremities back to the heart.

The Lymphatic System works to remove debris and other waste products. It is known as the sewer pipes of the body, because it carries away dead cells and other debris to be removed by the kidneys or the liver.

SIGNS OF PROBLEMS WITH YOUR CIRCULATION

Your feet will be one of the first places in your body to show visible signs of problems with your circulatory system. Here are some of the signs:

- Cool or cold skin temperature, especially in the feet.
- Lack of hair growth on the legs, feet and toes.
- Color changes in the foot to a more pinkish, purplish, or bluish hue.
- Leg cramps when you exercise.
- Pain in the feet or legs while lying in bed — the medical term is rest pain.

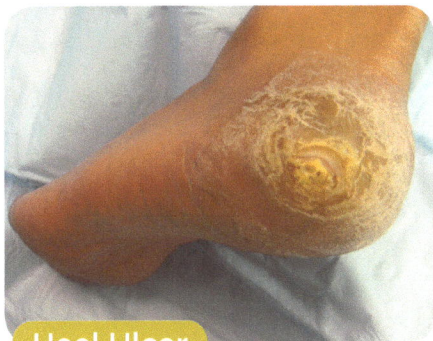

Heel Ulcer

- Pain or cramping in the calf or thigh when you walk a short distance — the medical term is intermittent claudication.
- Ulcers or wounds that are slow to heal or that do not heal.
- Absent or weak pulses in the feet or legs.

WHAT SKIN COLOR TELLS ABOUT YOU

The color of your skin can give you an indication about the issues you have related to circulation.

- **White or Grey:** Acute vascular occlusion is indicated.
- **Red:** A sign of early injury.
- **Purple:** Loss of adequate blood supply is indicated. The most common cause of the purple toe is from plaque being dislodged from large vessels and getting stuck in the smaller vessels in the toe.
- **Black:** Your tissue is dying and gangrene is present.

CARING FOR COLD FEET

- Wear one or two pairs of thick socks and warm house slippers.
- Wear thin silk socks under regular socks.

- Walk around.
- Do not warm your feet by using artificial heat sources such as heating pads, hot water bottles, or by sitting too close to a space heater, fireplace or campfire.

CARING FOR SWOLLEN FEET

Another sign of poor circulation is swelling, or edema, which is caused by fluid in the tissues of the leg and foot. Here are some things you can do to relieve swelling:

- Elevate your feet and legs. Use a foot stool, box, chair, recliner or foot rest. If you are on the couch, put your feet up on a pillow. Keep your feet above the level of your heart.

- Your doctor may advise you to take diuretics or water pills. If you take them, do so in the morning. These pills tend to make you urinate a lot, and that could interrupt your sleep if taken at bedtime. By having less fluid in your system, your blood pressure will be lowered.

- Your doctor may advise you to wear compression stockings. They keep adequate pressure on the leg so fluid won't collect. Be sure to put the stockings on before you get out of bed and before your legs start to swell.

- Press your finger to the skin on the bone along the front of your leg (the tibia). If there is an indentation after removing your finger, you have pitting edema. Heart or kidney problems or too much salt in your diet can cause this problem. See your primary care provider for an examination and treatment, and use less salt in your diet.

- Swelling in the legs from problems of the venous system can cause a complication to the skin called stasis dermatitis, which causes the skin to become dry and itchy. Scratching this vulnerable skin can result in a venous leg ulcer. You should be greatly helped by moisturizing lotions and compression stockings. The lotion keeps the skin supple and prevents dry and itchy skin and the compression stockings help prevent the accumulation of fluid in your legs.

DISEASES CAUSED BY POOR CIRCULATION

When your circulatory system doesn't function as it should,

your body is not getting an adequate blood supply, so your tissues may become damaged. Because this is a problem of your entire vascular system, you should have your organ systems checked. As far as your feet are concerned, you are at risk for infection, ulceration, and amputation.

Peripheral Arterial Disease

If there is blockage in your arteries, the term "PAD" or Peripheral Arterial Disease is used. If you have PAD, which means you are having problems with blood flow through your arteries to your extremities — arms and legs–and organs — like your heart, brain, and kidneys. This disease affects about eight to twelve million Americans, and most are over the age of fifty. Older, obese adults — women more than men — are especially prone to PAD.

You may have heard of the term "hardening of the arteries"— the medical term is atherosclerosis — which can cause heart attacks and strokes. PAD is a disease that affects your entire vascular system. Clogging in one area of the body indicates clogging is occurring in other parts of the body as well. This is why almost all those who have PAD in the feet and legs have problems with other organs.

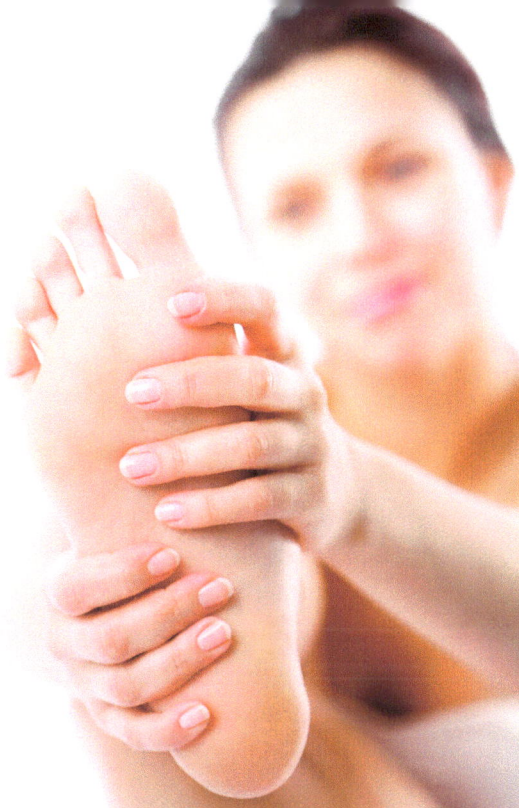

If you are suffering from aching in the legs, pain in the leg muscles, leg cramps or rest pain, and slow or non-healing ulcers, you may have PAD. These symptoms may come on silently in the early stages. There is one type of PAD for which there are no symptoms; which is termed asymptomatic.

You are at the highest risk for developing PAD if you are a former or current smoker, obese, and have a personal or family history of diabetes, kidney disease, high blood pressure, high cholesterol, or cardiovascular disease.

Peripheral Vascular Disease

Peripheral vascular disease (PVD) has been the name used for a multitude of circulatory problems that can affect the feet. The arteries may become narrow and hardened (athero-sclerosis), and are frequently blocked when cholesterol and scar tissue build up plaque inside the arteries.

Ischemia

The medical term for pain caused by the lack of circulation or blood flow to adequately maintain the tissues is ischemia. With ischemia, there is not enough oxygen or nutrients delivered to the tissue and there is a buildup of metabolic waste products. Ultimately, ischemia can lead to tissue death. Ischemia is often caused by a partial or total blockage of an artery.

Gangrene

Gangrene is death and decay of a body part due to deficiency of blood supply and is a frequent complication in the diabetic foot. Dry gangrene arises due to loss of blood supply from

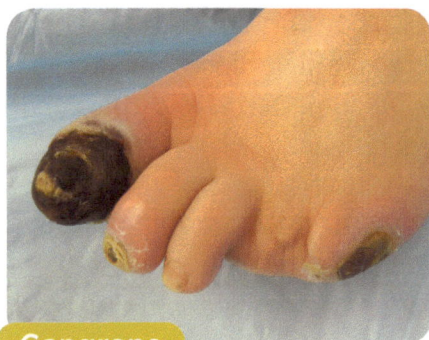

Gangrene

the artery; wet gangrene arises due to both the artery and the vein being blocked. Treatment for severe gangrene or ulcers that will not heal may include a bypass procedure to bring blood flow around a blocked artery, or a balloon angioplasty* and stenting* to restore blood flow in the lower extremities. Endovascular surgery is a relatively new procedure, which involves making an incision of less than one inch in the groin area to access the artery in the leg. A variety of micro instruments can then be inserted into the artery. A laser, for example, may be used to dissolve the plaque. Other instruments can remove the plaque or even open a new channel within the plaque to restore blood circulation to the foot.

Venous Insufficiency

Your blood travels back to your heart from your limbs and organs through two vein systems called the deep and superficial veins. If the valves of these veins are not working well — which

*balloon angioplasty: a technique that mechanically widens a narrow or obstructed blood vessel using a collapsed balloon on a guide wire, known as a balloon catheter.

*stenting: inserting an artificial tube into a natural passage in the body to prevent or avoid it from getting blocked or constricted.

may be caused by your lack of movement or chronic standing — you may develop a disease of the veins called venous insufficiency. The result is that fluid leaks out of the veins into the tissues and the leg will swell. The medical term for swelling is edema. If you have this problem, your skin will likely become dry, inflamed and itchy. But, if you scratch your legs, you can complicate an already bad situation by causing the area to ulcerate. These sores or lesions can become large and extremely difficult to heal.

If you have venous insufficiency, you should see a vascular specialist for treatment. This might involve tying off a small vein that connects the deep to the superficial system, using compression stockings, applying an absorbent dressing or wearing a compression boot using pneumatic medicine.

DIAGNOSING CIRCULATORY PROBLEMS

There are a number of diagnostic tests available to identify the location and extent of your circulatory problems. Imaging of the arterial system is necessary to determine if your foot issues — such as pain while resting, non-healing foot ulcers, or impaired gait — are a result of reduced

FACTS

Poor circulation is caused by plaque, made from fats such as cholesterol and triglycerides, which build up and harden in your arteries, and may block the blood supply to your foot.

blood supply to your leg muscles. This information helps the vascular surgeon decide what type of treatment may be best for you.

When your health care provider is examining you for a foot wound that won't heal, your circulation should be tested. A safe and reliable test used to measure circulation in the leg is an Ankle Brachial Index (ABI) with Segmental Pressures Test. It involves inflating a series of blood pressure cuffs and measuring the blood flow in your leg, foot, and toes, and comparing those measurements to the blood flow in your arm. This test may help the vascular specialist determine whether you have vascular disease due to diabetes and PAD. In addition to identifying whether there is a problem with the circulation, it can reveal the location in the foot or leg where the circulation is decreased or absent, as well as where the body has sufficient circulation to heal the wound if amputation is necessary.

Another more specific test is called an arteriogram. This test requires the injection of a dye into an artery, followed by a series of X-rays that track the progress of the dye as it moves down the leg toward the foot. Blocked or narrowed arteries can be pinpointed on the X-rays.

Yet another test that evaluates the vascular system or blood vessels is called magnetic resonance angiogram or MRA. This relatively new test is non-invasive, fast and easy and does not involve catheters, radiation, or the use of contrast materials. With this technique, your entire vascular system — from your abdominal aorta to your foot — can be viewed in less than two minutes.

Sometimes, problems with your legs are the first sign of circulatory concerns. Vascular testing can also identify whether other systems are simultaneously being affected by vascular disease. This is critical because circulatory problems can have serious complications such as a stroke, blood clots, or heart attack.

POOR CIRCULATION IMPACTS HEALING OF FOOT WOUNDS

Proper circulation is essential for a foot wound to heal. Without it, tissue dies. The circulatory system in the leg is a "closed" system, which means that there is no way to get more blood flow into it, until you get some out of it. No fresh, oxygenated blood that carries nutrients, and medications can get to a foot wound until some blood containing carbon dioxide and metabolic waste products is moved back toward the heart. Your body should be able to heal wounds from minor traumas, such as a blister or a cut. But if your circulation is impaired, you will have a more difficult time healing a foot wound like an infection or ulcer. Some people's foot wounds will not heal because their circulation is so poor.

TREATMENT FOR POOR CIRCULATION

Helping your circulatory system work better is your job. The easiest and most cost effective method of increasing your circulation is to change your behavior: stop smoking, start an exercise program, eat healthy foods in reasonable portions, keep your blood sugar levels in the normal range and see your health care provider regularly. Your doctor may reccomend treatment in the form of medication to help prevent platelets from clustering together to form a blood clot.

DISEASES CAUSED BY POOR CIRCULATION

Peripheral Artery Disease

Peripheral Vascular Disease

Ischemia

Gangrene

Venous Insufficiency

CHAPTER 15
INFECTIONS &
INFLAMMATION

"Cherish your health: If it is good, preserve it. If is unstable, improve it. If it is beyond what you can improve, get help."

— George Carlin

People with diabetes who have high blood sugars most of the time are more likely to develop infections than people with normal blood sugars. People with diabetes who do not practice good hygiene are also the most vulnerable to infections.

The good news is that there is a lot that you can do to prevent getting an infection. The bad news is that if you do get an infection and it is not attended to promptly, it can be the start of a difficult treatment process, which could go as far as requiring an amputation.

In general, foot infections in persons with diabetes become more severe and take longer to cure than do the same infections in persons without diabetes.

Foot infections account for the largest number of diabetes-related hospital admissions and are the most common non-traumatic cause of amputations. If left untreated, these infections can threaten life and limb.

GOOD HYGIENE

If you have read this entire book, you may have seen these recommendations before. However, they are being repeated here as a reminder that tending to your foot health is critical to prevent infections, get rid of infections, prevent recurrence of infections and to avoid picking up new infections.

If you practice these preventive foot health behaviors, the chances of developing a problem will be minimal.

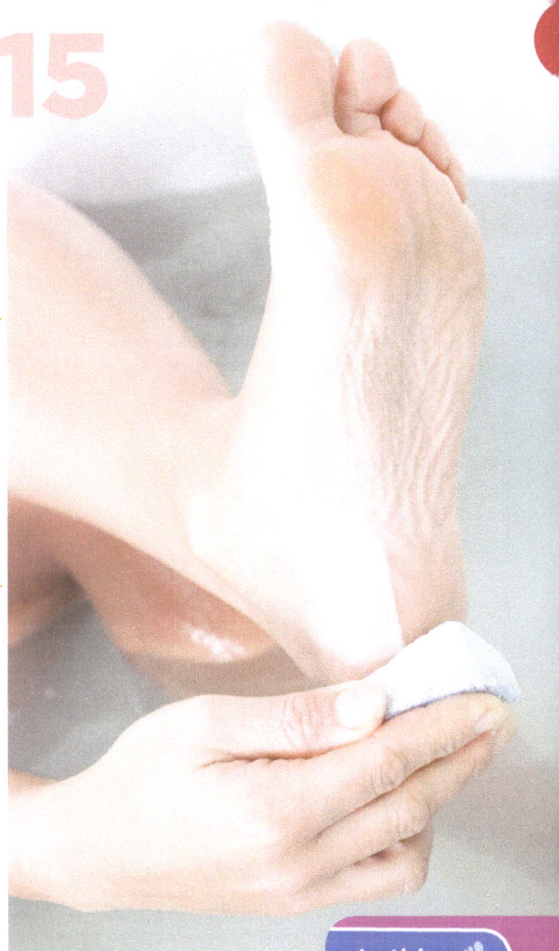

Here are some tips to prevent infections:

Do's

- Bathe your feet everyday.

- Keep wounds covered.

- Sterilize linens.

- Wash your hands often.

- Use an antibacterial cleaner like Lysol™ to keep surfaces clean and to clean your shoes. If you can't clean your shoes, replace them.

Don'ts

- Don't share items used for your personal hygiene: towels, shoes, socks, make-up, or other toiletries.

- Don't think running soapy water OVER your feet in the shower MEANS CLEANING your feet. You must actually wash the feet and in between the toes with soap. Rinse your feet well, and gently pat them dry, paying particular attention to the areas between the toes.

- Don't put on a sock or shoe that is damp from perspiration or from exposure to wet conditions.

- Don't mistake a skin infection for dry skin. If you've been using lotion regularly and your dry, scaly skin persists, see a foot care specialist to check for an infection.

You will identify problems early and resolve them promptly.

Inspecting your feet everyday is the most cost-effective way to prevent foot infections and reduce your health care costs. Exercise, proper nutrition, and smoking cessation, which are important in diabetes care in general, are also important in preventing foot ulcers.

TIPS FOR GOOD FOOT HYGIENE

- Inspect your feet daily, especially between your toes, for sores or cuts. If you cannot see your foot directly, use a mirror on the floor or a long handled mirror. If you cannot see your feet, ask your caregiver to check them every day. Any changes, even small ones, should be evaluated.

- A locally red, swollen, or warm area on your foot should prompt you to call your physician or foot care specialist for an evaluation.

- Bathe your feet daily, using soap and water. Check the temperature of the bath water with your hand, elbow or thermometer.

- Use a clean towel to dry your feet thoroughly, especially between the toes. A hair

Inspect your feet daily, especially between your toes, for sores or cuts.

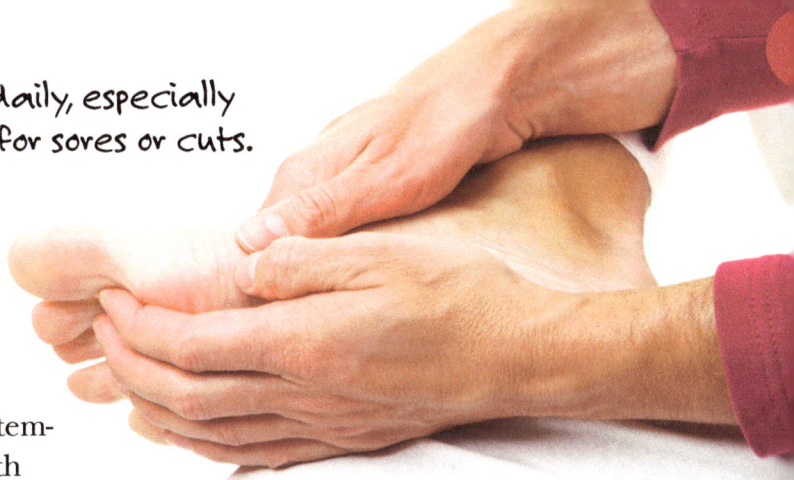

dryer set on the coolest temperature can be used with caution, and use powder if necessary after drying.

- Wear well-fitted, clean socks every day.
- Wear shoes at all times. Don't walk barefooted or just with socks. Use shoes around the house, clogs in the shower, swim sneakers at the pool.
- Be sure your shoes are fitted properly to avoid friction or pressure. Inspect shoes daily for foreign objects or irregularities such as loose stitching that can cause foot wounds.
- Use lotion on your legs and feet to avoid dryness and cracking of the skin.
- Trim toenails with the contour of the toe. File rough or sharp edges with an emery board.

TREATING INFECTIONS: WHAT YOU CAN DO

If you have a superficial skin infection, your podiatrist can give you a surgical scrub brush and antibacterial soap to use as the best way to insure foot hygiene.

You should wash, rinse and dry your feet well, and apply a topical anti-fungal powder or cream if appropriate.

If you have an infection caused by a bacteria named pseudomonas, your wound will have an odor similar to a gymnasium or old athletic shoes. To kill the pseudomonas bacteria, your doctor will use a combination of topical and oral antibiotics and a local treatment for the foot. You can help by mixing half a cup of white vinegar (a dilute acid) in a pan of room temperature tap water and soak your foot in this solution for twenty minutes twice a day.

If your infection is between your toes, soak a piece of cotton or gauze in the vinegar solution described above and put it between your toes to help kill the bacteria, or place the cotton or gauze between the toes while soaking. This separates the toes and assures the solution is reaching all of the infected skin.

It is also very important to keep your home environment clean. You should use Lysol™, bleach, or an antibacterial cleaner. Foot infections get passed from person-to-person at home when the infected person walks barefooted in the house, leaving bacteria or fungus on the floor for family or friends to pick up through an opening or a crack in their feet. Germs can also live in a shower, bathtub or swimming pool.

SIGNS OF INFLAMMATION

Redness

Swelling

Heat

Pain

LOSS OF PROTECTIVE SENSATION FOR PAIN

(See Chapter 12 on Nerve Damage) If you have diabetes and do not feel pain in your feet, you may have sensory neuropathy, and, as such, you should be even more vigilant when it comes to infections. If you experience a trauma to your foot, you may not feel it, it may be "silent" or painless. So, you may have no idea that you have been injured or that you have an infection. Just because you do not have pain does not mean that you do not have a problem. Nothing could be further from the truth. If you do not visually examine your foot, you may not realize that you have an infection until you see blood or pus on your socks. The sooner you get treatment for an infection, the better your chances are of keeping it under control. If you wait too long, you are putting your foot at risk.

YOUR IMMUNE SYSTEM

You can't feel it or see it, but your immune system is quietly and constantly patrolling your body to detect and destroy infectious microbes. It is your most powerful protector, working tirelessly around-the-clock to keep you safe and healthy. Your immune system fights and removes infections from your body, defending it against infectious disease and foreign materials. Its "soldiers" are white blood cells or leukocytes, produced in the bone marrow, whose job is to kill bacteria.

A person with a weakened immune system, or immunopathy, doesn't have the same ability to heal a wound or fight infection. Deficiencies in the immune system not only leave the body more vulnerable to infections, but also create problems that can complicate healing.

Most wound care specialists believe that because the immune system of people with diabetes is compromised, the wound fails to heal because it is stuck in the inflammatory phase of healing. As a result, there is the potential for a long, drawn-out fight between the forces that heal wounds and infections and those that complicate and delay the healing process.

As you age, you also become more vulnerable. Researchers believe that the aging process somehow leads to a reduction of immune response capability, which in turn contributes to more infections and inflammatory diseases. While some people age healthily, the elderly are far more likely to contract infectious diseases. Respiratory infections, influenza, and particularly pneumonia are a leading cause of death in people over sixty-five worldwide.

Healthy living strategies are the best way to give your immune system the upper hand. Following general good-health guidelines is the single best step you can take toward keeping your immune system strong and healthy. Every part of your body, including your immune system, functions better when protected from environmental assaults and bolstered by healthy living strategies.

INFLAMMATION

When you have an infection, an irritation or a similar type of trauma, it will often cause inflammation. You know there is inflammation when you see redness and swelling and feel heat and pain to the site of the problem. This is actually a good thing. Swelling helps by diluting any irritants in the injured area, bringing proteins (called fibrinogens) to form a mesh to cover the wound, trapping foreign particles, and forming the foundation for new tissue to be laid down to enhance the effectiveness of the immune system.

TYPES OF INFECTIONS

Bacterial Infections

If you have a bacterial infection, it means that bacteria have penetrated your skin — the protective envelope that covers your body. Most infections start off as mild infections, but also have the potential to become serious. Foot infections often start out small and are relatively easy to treat, like an ingrown toenail or an area of damaged tissue that may have a small collection of pus in the tissues, called an abscess, confined to one area.

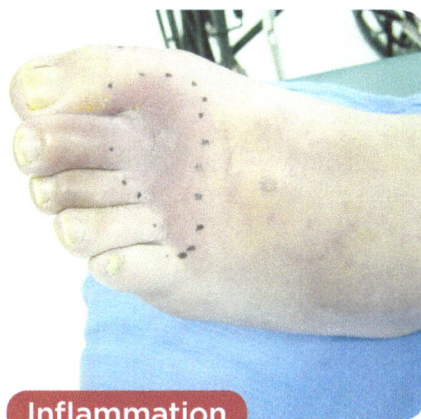

Inflammation

✓

**WOUND
EVALUATION**

Width

Length

Depth

Color

Skin
Condition

Odor

If you suspect you have a foot infection, see a foot care professional. The doctor can then evaluate the wound and determine its size, the condition of the tissues, and what vital structures may be affected. It is important to first determine the cause of the infection and the extent of the wound so that it can be appropriately treated. For example, if you have an ulcer, your wound may have to be probed to see if it extends to the underlying bone. The doctor will determine the severity of the wound by measuring its width, length, and depth, and by evaluating the condition of the wound in terms of color, skin condition, and whether the wound has an odor. A tissue sample may be taken to send to a pathologist to be analyzed. This helps to determine which antibiotics are needed.

There can be, and usually are, multiple species of bacteria in a chronic or longstanding wound, and a different antibiotic may be needed to treat different bacteria. The idea is to find the antibiotic with the highest potency to kill the infection at the lowest dosage. This is called the Minimum Inhibitory Concentration (MIC). When your doctor identifies the specific bacteria causing the problem, he or she can choose the antibiotic

that would be most effective. A preliminary test on the tissue specimen sent to the lab is called a Gram stain.

Another test that must be performed on this tissue is a Culture and Sensitivity (C & S) Test, which should take one to two days to complete. These tests help the doctor decide which antibiotic would be best and which method would be most appropriate to give you the antibiotic: by mouth (oral); on the skin (topical); through your veins (intravenous) or by injection into a muscle (intra-muscular). The method of giving you the antibiotics may also depend on the antibiotic itself. Your doctor will take into consideration other medications you may be taking or any allergies to medications you may have, to prevent any possible interactions with the antibiotic being considered.

For example, if you have a fever, an elevated white cell count, and an elevated sedimentation rate, you need to get antibiotics in your body quickly. The fastest way is through a vein (intravenous) followed by injecting it into a muscle (intramuscular), usually in the arm or the buttocks. There are some antibiotics, though, that can only be given intravenously no matter what your condition.

Unfortunately, some bacteria

have become increasingly resistant to antibiotics that are used to treat foot wounds and infections, so the choice for antibiotics is becoming more difficult. If you are told that you have Methicillin Resistant Staphylococcus Aureus or MRSA, it means that the bacteria you have acquired is more resistant to treatment. In the past, MRSA was acquired only in a hospital; however, today, it is frequently acquired in the community and other healthcare facilities. Follow the "top tips" (on page 92) to prevent acquiring this bacteria in public places.

MOST INFECTIONS START OFF AS MILD, BUT HAVE THE POTENTIAL TO BECOME SERIOUS.

FACTS

Bone infections

Osteomyelitis most commonly occurs in the foot when bacteria gain access to the bone from a nearby or close by or contiguous soft tissue infection or foot ulcer. Early detection of osteomyelitis is very important both to limit the destruction of the bone and to stand a better chance of re-

solving the infection with antibiotics rather than surgery.

A bone infection is the most-feared foot complication for a person with diabetes. If you are being aggressively treated for a foot wound and it does not heal in six weeks, your doctor will likely want to examine the underlying bone for infection. If a bone infection is suspected, an X-ray or magnetic resonance imaging (MRI) or bone scan will be performed to diagnose any infection as early as possible.

Osteomyelitis in the diabetic foot can lead to life-threatening complications, such as limb loss or even blood poisoning, known as septecemia. So, getting a proper diagnosis and timely treatment is vital.

Mold, Yeast & Fungus Infections: Dermatophytes

The dark, moist, and warm environment inside your shoe is the perfect place for mold, yeast and fungus to prosper. Infections caused by these troublemakers

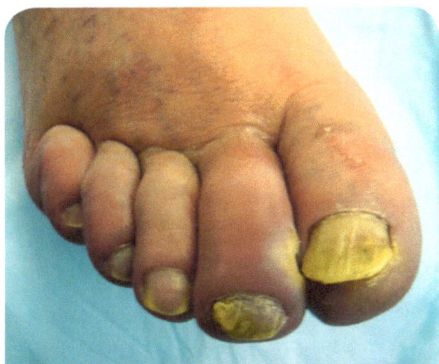

2nd Toe With Osteomyelitis

and adding KOH (potassium hydroxide) to help review the specimen under a microscope. A fungal culture involves taking a specimen of the affected skin and submitting it for anatomical pathology or PAS testing, a more sensitive test for determining if you have a mold, yeast, or fungus infection.

Once the diagnosis has been confirmed, treatment involves better hygiene, oral and or topical medications, switching from a closed shoe to a surgical shoe, cleaning the environment where you may have stood barefooted, and cleaning the wound (debridment) as necessary to reduce the amount of dead tissue, called bioburden, your body needs to deal with when you have an infection.

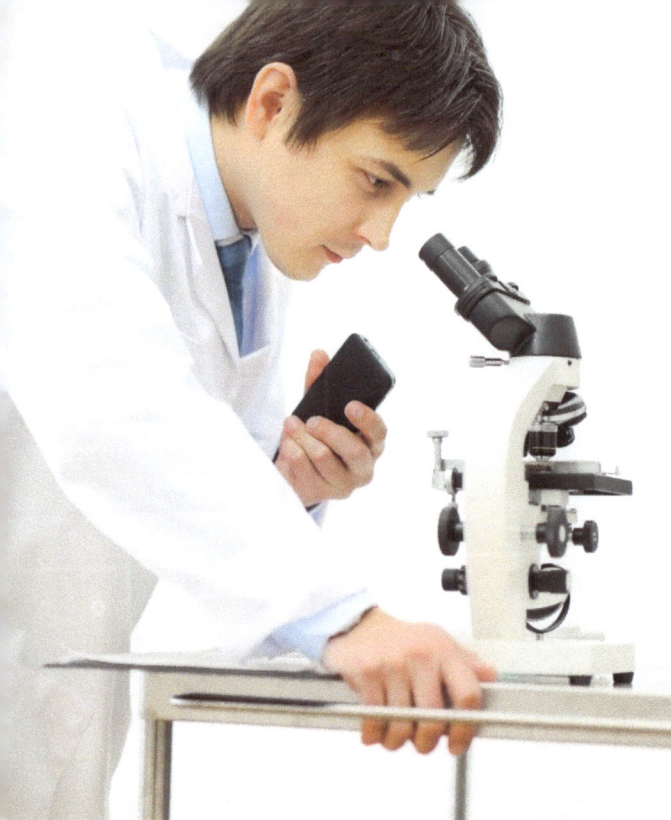

may occur on your nails, between your toes, or on the sides or bottom of your foot. They are usually responsible for superficial skin infections on your foot often referred to as tinea pedis or "athlete's foot."

If you notice whitish, inflamed, itchy, and peeling skin on the foot, you may think you just have dry skin, but you may have a mold, yeast or fungal infection. Do not scratch this itch, because the infection can spread to other parts of your body via your hands.

Diagnosis & Treatment

Treatment depends on the proper diagnosis. There are several ways to diagnose this problem. A KOH test involves placing a scraping of tissue on a slide

Mixed Bacterial and Fungal Infection

People who have infections over a time period of several weeks to months often have a mixed bacterial and fungal infection. Once either bacteria or fungal organisms have invaded the skin, they can be infected with any other organisms with which they come into contact. The diagnosis and treatment will be the same; however, your doctor should perform the appropriate testing to identify all of the organisms in your wound. Since there are both oral and topical medications that can be used, you can expect a combination of therapies to be used to cure your infection.

Viral Infections

In addition to a bacterial infection, your feet may also be subject to a viral infection. The most commonly seen viral infection is a wart (the medical term is verruca). Warts are part of the human papilloma virus family. They are parasites that take nourishment and oxygen from your body and excrete metabolic waste products into your body. Warts are infectious critters.

If you have a wart, see a foot care professional for treatment. DO NOT use an over-the-counter product designed for treating warts. Unfortunately, these products contain salicylic acid and cause chemical burns, destroy tissue painlessly and become a trigger that has the potential to lead to major foot problem, including an amputation.

Gout/Inflammation

There is a close relationship between Type 2 diabetes (diabetes mellitus) and gout. Each disorder may be guilty of triggering the other. Some studies have shown that gout sufferers have a higher risk of developing Type 2 diabetes in later life, while others have found that gout sometimes develops in people already suffering from diabetes. When gout is caused by diabetes, it is often referred to as "secondary gout" and usually occurs in elderly people. This doesn't mean that if you have diabetes, that gout is definitely going to be part of your future. But, you should be on the lookout for gout symptoms — pain, swelling, redness, heat, and stiffness. Better yet, you can take some preventative steps to avoid getting this disorder.

Gout is caused by high levels of uric acid building up in the extremities and joints of the body; in the foot, this typically impacts the big toe joint and ankles. Uric acid crystals with sharp points are deposited in the joints, which results in inflammation. Some people with gout have pain and functional disability; others have skin wounds

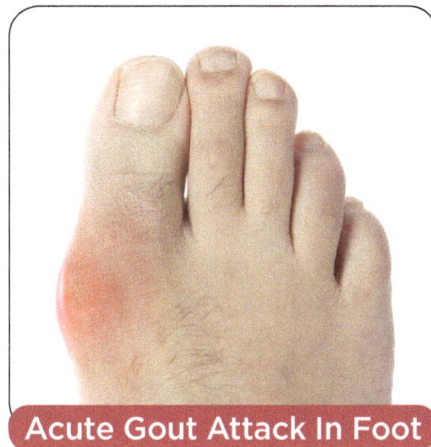

Acute Gout Attack In Foot

from where the uric acid crystals are literally "escaping" through the soft tissue. In any case, it is a painful disorder and can cause a form of arthritis called gouty arthropathy.

If you have diabetes and hope to prevent gout, you should follow a sensible, healthy diet; exercise; and cut out alcohol. Exercise will help improve the circulation of blood around your body and prevent the build up of uric acid. You should stay away from foods containing purines, most often found in red meat, organ meat, beer, wine, and liquor (clear spirits gin or vodka may be acceptable). In fact, modifying your diet to limit purine intake will almost always control your uric acid levels. Other preventative measures include drinking plenty of water. Check with your medical practitioner about a medication named Allopurinol™ or using herbal remedies such as cayenne tincture and gingko biloba. With your cooperation, gout is almost 100 percent preventable.

STATISTICS

The dangers of infection are very real; infections are the eighth leading cause of death in the United States. Every year, 60,000 people in the United States die from pneumonia. About 215,000 people die from a severe bacterial infection known as sepsis, which is more than the number who die from breast, colorectal, pancreatic, and prostate cancers combined. Tuberculosis, once considered under control, was responsible for 1.7 million deaths in 2004. At the same time, infectious diseases are emerging around the globe in such forms as bird flu and severe acute respiratory syndrome (SARS).

Other preventative measures include drinking plenty of water.

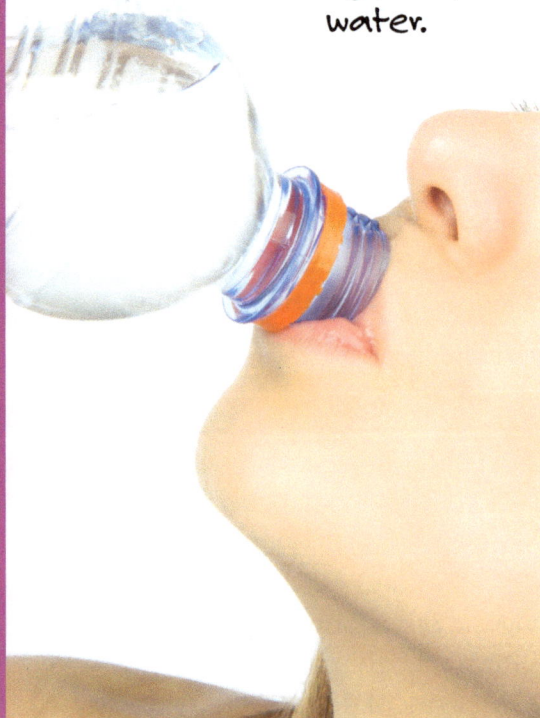

ULCERS

And I came close to losing a part of my foot on two occasions. I hope I'm consistently lucky and that the next time I develop a blister or step on something sharp, that I don't go as far as I did on those two times.

— **Mary Tyler Moore**

A foot ulcer is an open sore, wound or hole somewhere on your foot; a crater-shaped break in the skin. It often occurs in high-pressure areas — under or around a corn or callus. The break may appear to be small, but a larger ulcer may be hidden under the skin growth or keratosis. Up to 82 percent of foot ulcers are related to pressure from footwear or narrow or otherwise inadequate or improperly fitted footwear. Foot ulcers can be caused by painless or silent trauma from mechanical, chemical, or thermal trauma. *(See Chapter 12)*

Once you've had an ulcer, you are more likely to get another one, because you have had serious damage to the nerves and blood vessels of your feet and because getting an ulcer is usually a sign that you are not taking good care of your feet.

In this chapter

PREVENTION

LOCATIONS

TREATMENT

SOLUTIONS

PREVENTING FOOT ULCERS

All the steps you have been told to heed in taking care of your feet are very important to all people with diabetes, because foot ulcers can be avoided.

Here are a few reminders:

1. Control your blood sugar levels
2. Don't smoke or use tobacco products
3. Control your weight
4. Inspect your feet every day

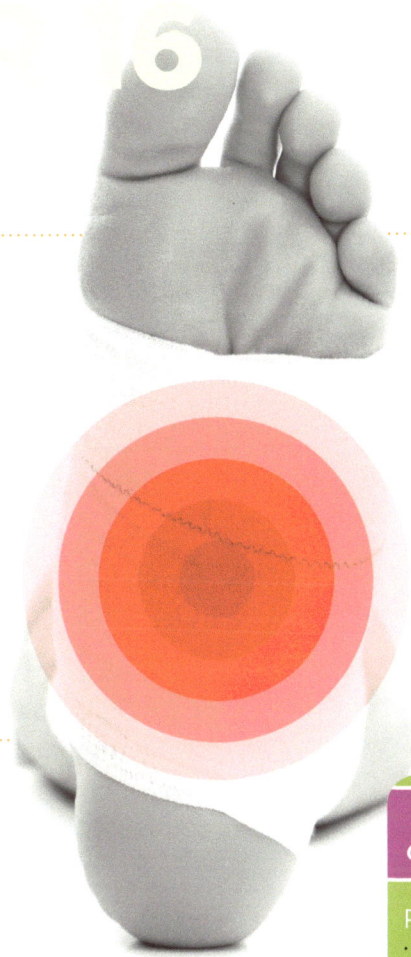

5. Keep your feet dry and clean.

6. Wear well-fitted shoes and socks.

7. Don't go barefoot.

8. Don't soak your feet.

9. Don't put lotion between your toes.

10. Put lotion on the rest of your foot.

11. Have an annual foot exam that includes a monofilament test.

12. See a foot specialist to treat corns, calluses, toenails or any injury or condition of your foot.

COMMON LOCATIONS OF FOOT ULCERS

The parts of the foot that receive the highest stress, friction, force or pressure are the most likely to ulcerate. A pressure-mapping machine can analyze your gait and show where the highest forces are on the bottom of your foot when you walk across it.

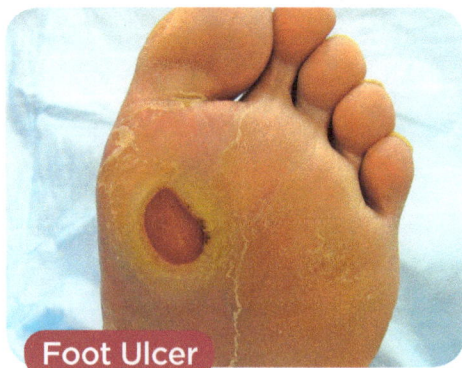

Foot Ulcer

- Ulcers on the top of the toes are due to deformed toes interacting with shoes that fit poorly. Changing shoes to a deeper and wider toe box can prevent re-ulceration.

- Ulcers on the bottom of the foot are due more to pressure and friction issues. Reducing pressure and friction by offloading the site of the ulcer with accommodative pads or biomechanical orthotics and a variety of other methods can prevent recurrent ulcers.

- The back and bottom of the heel has a small surface space to absorb a large about of pressure. Ulcers generated by pressure or friction where bed sheets rub against the foot are usually seen in people with diabetes who are bedridden for long time periods. Because of their location and the fragility of the tissues in that location, heel ulcers often require substantial treatment.

Treatment

Foot ulcers should be treated by professionals. Your foot care specialist will determine the cause of your ulcer by taking your history, performing a physical exam, and evaluating your circulation and nerves. Bacterial cultures may be taken to identify the organism causing the infections and X-rays should be taken to see if there is an infection of the bones and to assure that the proper therapy — including local care and antibiotics — can be prescribed. The ulcer can be trimmed and dead tissue can be cut away (de-brided); the appropriate dress-ings applied, and a surgical shoe prescribed. Most importantly, your foot care specialist will cre-ate a treatment plan for healing your foot ulcer and preventing a re-occurrence.

Here are some things you can do to recover more quickly:

- Follow your treatment plan instructions.

- Keep your wound clean and dry, covered with a bandage.

- Inspect your wound daily.

- Wear the surgical shoe prescribed.

- Buy new shoes (if needed).

- After the wound is healed, use the proper foot gear to prevent another ulcer. Special diabetic or custom molded shoes and insoles may be best.

- Stay off your foot (bed rest, crutches, or a wheelchair may be prescribed).

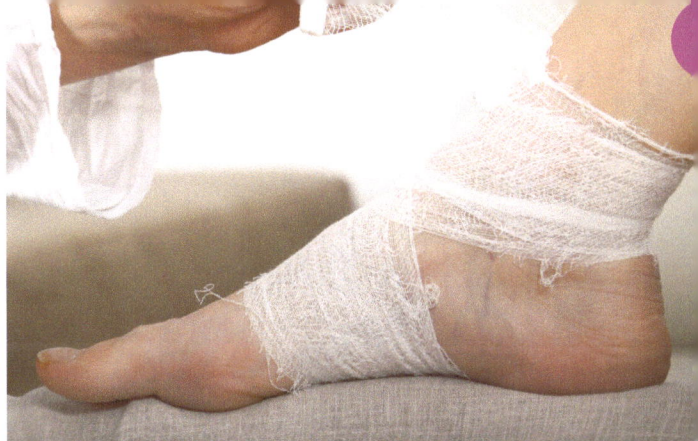

ULCER TREATMENT

Healing a foot ulcer is much like solving a puzzle. Ulcers are com-plex wounds. Understanding the reason the ulcer has developed is important in determining how to treat it. Usually, there are mul-tiple contributing factors. If each of these factors has not been identified and treated correctly, the ulcer could fail to heal. If the ulcer does not heal, it is a very serious threat to the foot and could even result in an amputa-tion. Even if it does heal, it can still return.

Getting a foot ulcer to heal takes great patience, meticulous care and great expense. The fol-lowing are several steps involved:

Cleaning the Ulcer: Debridement

The primary goal for the care of a foot ulcer is to get it to close up as quickly as possible. But first, it must be cleaned. There are vari-ous types of debridement:

- **Autolytic:** (healing which occurs naturally on its own), mechanical, enzymatic,

sharp/surgical, and biosurgical

- **Mechanical debridement** is usually accomplished with a dry dressing or whirlpool.

- **Enzymatic debridement** involves the topical application of a debriding enzyme to the wound.

- **Surgical debridement** involves surgically removing dead tissue regularly. Because reducing the amount of dead tissue in the wound, called bioburden, expedites healing, it increases the probability of the wound closing fully.

- **Biosurgical debridement** includes surgery systems that use specialized water jet-powered surgical tools designed to cut and remove unwanted tissue from ulcers or wounds.

- **Ultrasonic debridement** is a relatively new and virtually pain-free way to clean wounds. These devices are safe, efficient and offer rapid results.

- **Polyacrylate debriding** systems are a quick, simple, safe, and pain-free dressing that provides 24-hour simultaneous rinsing and debriding. The dressing is only changed once per day, and families can be taught to handle it as part of home care. The dressing provides constant cleaning of the wound.

- **Negative Pressure Wound Therapy (NPWT)** promotes wound healing by applying a vacuum through a specially-sealed dressing. The continued vacuum draws out fluid from the wound and increases blood flow to the area. A popular product in the field is KCI Wound V.A.C. (kci1.com/KCI1/vactherapy)

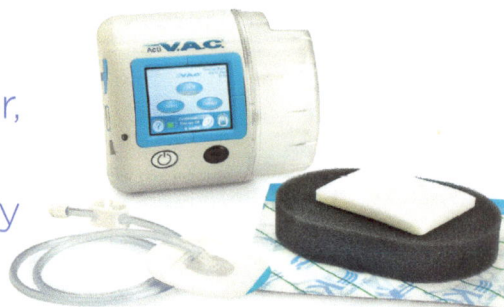

FACTS

At any given time, approximately 5 percent of the diabetic population will have a foot ulcer, and almost half of them are infected by the time medical attention is sought.

SOLUTIONS TO OFFLOAD-ING & REDISTRIBUTING PRESSURE

About 90 percent of foot ulcers develop because of abnormal pressure, friction, and stress against the foot. Offloading and reducing the abnormal forces against the foot are critical to preventing diabetic ulcers and do many positive things:

- Reduce shock and shear forces

- Cushion the foot

- Redistribute plantar pressure

- Realign mechanically imbal-anced structures to permit a wound to heal

If you have an ulcer, it is important that the solution is tailored to your lifestyle. The goal is to help you stay mobile while preventing excessive pres-sure to the wound. However, you must commit to wearing the offloading device at all times, even during trips to the bath-room at night.

Some of the options you may be given include a:

- Pad
- Insole
- Shoe
- Crutch
- Boot
- Walker

People with a history of a diabetic foot ulcer have a 40% greater 10 year mortality than people with diabetes alone.

FACTS

- Wheelchair

- Scooter

- Bed rest

- Limited walking

- A removable walking cast

- Custom-molded prescription orthotics can be used within a surgical shoe during the healing phase.

- Roller Aid, an assistive device made of tubular aluminum that has wheels on the bottom.

- Total Contact Cast (TCC) or a full-contact cast: a piece of particle board or plywood placed across the bottom of the foot with a cast that cov-ers everything so that when you stand, all the weight is dispersed equally over the wood surface. A 21st century version of a Total Contact Cast is now available at Med Efficiency, Inc. (www.medefficiency.com)

- Walking boot

Full chamber total body hyperbaric oxygen also has

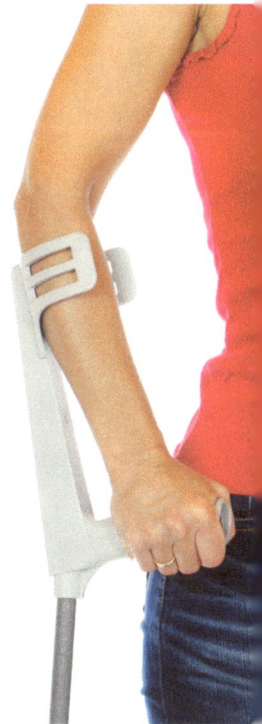

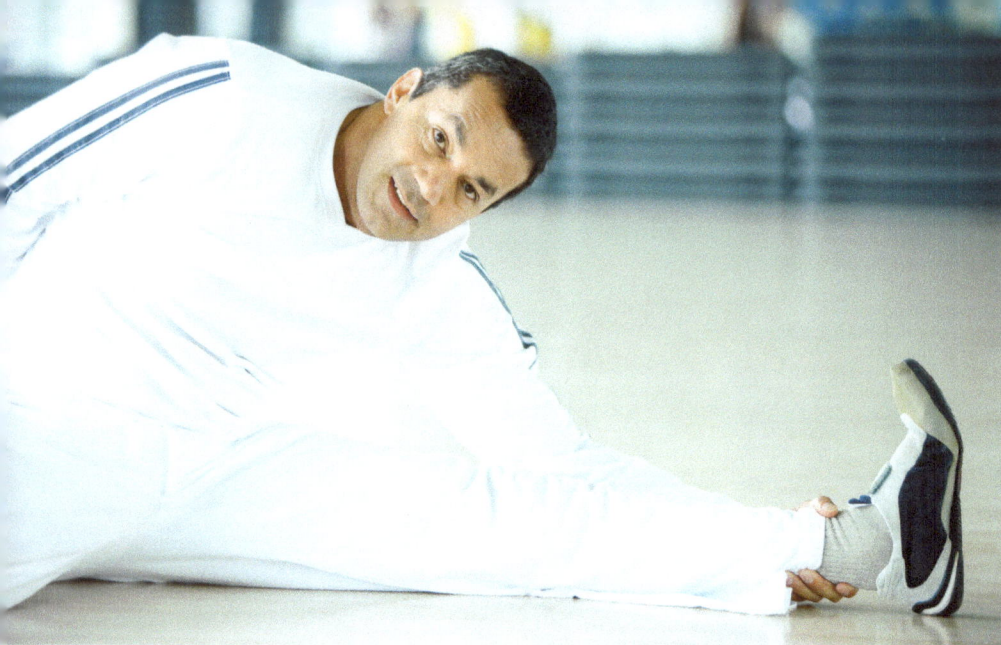

About 15-25 percent of people with diabetes will have a foot ulcer at least once in their lifetime. Most — about 70% — will heal with basic foot care. However, a foot ulcer can escalate quickly into a significant problem if an infection occurs. To resolve it may require hospitalization, intravenous antibiotics and perhaps even vascular surgery or surgery to remove infected tissue to avoid an amputation.

proven helpful in the treatment of lower extremity wounds from a variety of causes.

FOOT SUGERY TO AVOID ULCERS

If you have an ulcer, you may benefit by having foot surgery. Here are some things to consider:

- Surgery could be done to correct a foot problem before it can cause an infection or ulcer.

- Reconstructive Surgery may be considered when treating a non-healing or recurrent ulcer that is caused by a bone problem that cannot be treated in a conservative manner with a pad or brace.

- Opening a deep abscess and cleaning out infected or dead tissue could help cure your problem

- A partial or total foot amputation may be necessary.

PREVENTING RECURRENCE

If you have a history of foot ulcers, you are at high risk for ulcer recurrence. Re-ulceration can be prevented; however, in order to do so, you must invest time and effort in working with your foot care specialist and primary healthcare provider.

You will need to commit to regular risk and biomechanical assessments, tight glycemic control, to stop smoking, diet, exercise, and perhaps to wearing custom-molded orthotics and specialized supportive footwear and/or insoles, as well as practicing preventive foot care behaviors.

RISK OF RE-ULCERATION

The most common issues that impact on re-ulceration include:

- Being male
- Being older than sixty
- Having Type-2 diabetes
- Having diabetes longer than 10 years
- Alcohol abuse
- Tobacco abuse
- Nephropathy (kidney disease)
- Retinopathy (eye disease of retina)
- Neuropathy (nervous system disease)

FACTS

MORE THAN HALF OF ALL FOOT ULCERS (WOUNDS) WILL BECOME INFECTED, REQUIRING HOSPITALIZATION AND 1 IN 5 WILL REQUIRE AN AMPUTATION.

- Peripheral Vascular Disease (circulatory problems)
- Having a history of amputation
- Having elevated pressure on foot
- Having a rigid toe deformity or Charcot foot
- Having extra pressure on the bottom of the foot from prominent or abnormally shaped sesamoid bones under the big toe

SIGNS OF INFECTION

- Redness
- Swelling
- Increased warmth
- Pain, tenderness, limited motion to affected part
- Pus, drainage from wound
- Fever, chills, high blood pressure combined with elevated blood sugars (This means

that your infection has spread beyond the wound; go to the Emergency Room immediately.)

POOR CIRCULATION: PERIPHERAL ARTERIAL DISEASE (PAD) AND ITS IMPACT ON ULCERS

Peripheral artery disease (PAD) is caused by the accumulation of fatty deposits known as plaque in the arteries. The plaque restricts blood flow to the extremities and organ systems. PAD is one of the main complications of diabetes. When you have poor circulation and develop a foot ulcer, you are at greater risk of having an amputation.

✓

SIGNS OF INFECTION

Redness

Swelling

Increased warmth

Pus

Fever, chills, high blood pressure combinesd with elevated blood sugar

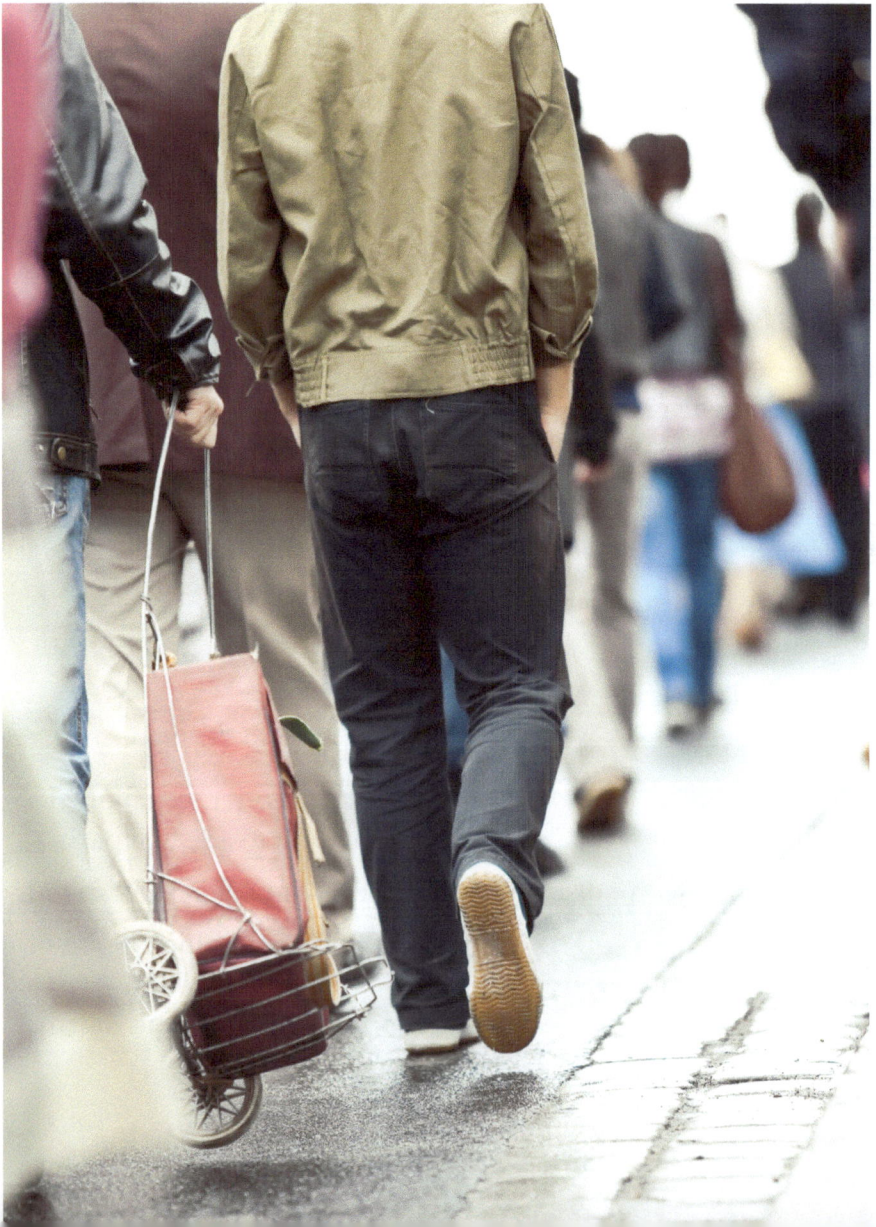

CHAPTER 17
AMPUTATION

*If I had known this was
going to happen to me,
I would have taken
better care of myself*

— Patient with diabetes

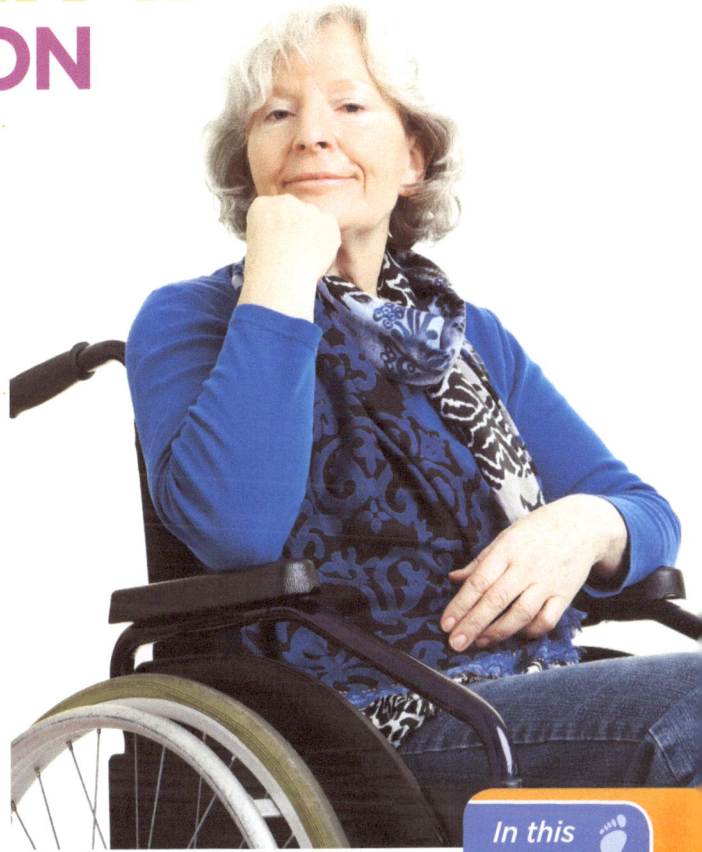

Foot or leg amputation could happen to you. This book has been dedicated to getting you to take better care of yourself so that you don't have to worry about what we are going to discuss in this chapter. But, unfortunately, 10 percent of people with diabetes do have an amputation. In fact, diabetes is the leading cause of non-traumatic lower extremity amputations. Toe and partial foot amputations are common.

Amputation rates are greater with increasing age, in males compared with females, and among African and Hispanic Americans.

More than half of those could have been prevented by good blood sugar control, better preventive foot care and better care of foot ulcers.

WHEN IS AN AMPUTATION NECESSARY?

If you have practiced preventive behaviors, followed your physician's recommendations for treating your wound or infection on your feet, and, yet, you continue to have pain or worse, and you have a non-painful wound that is infected and won't heal, you may need an amputation. That is because a non-healing wound or infection that may spread and can actually cause a more serious a life-threatening complication that is even worse than losing a part of your foot or your leg. There are several scenarios that may leave a person no choice except to lose a leg.

There are some cases where an amputation IS the most appropriate course of action. Your

In this chapter

WHEN IT IS NECESSARY

COUNSELING

REMAINING LEG

LIVING WITH AN AMPUTATION

medical team may recommend that you have an amputation if:

- You are not willing to undergo what could be multiple surgeries to treat your current infection and the post-operative rehabilitation. Your surgeon will explain that those surgeries, like all surgical procedures, are not guaranteed to bring the desired results.

- You may not be healthy enough to endure the rigors of wound healing.

- Your limb, if it can be salvaged, may leave you with an unstable biomechanical "platform" on which to stand, so that an amputation might actually require less time and rehabilitation toward resuming your activities of daily living.

PSYCHOLOGICAL COUNSELING

Every person undergoing an amputation should have the benefit of psychological counseling both before and after surgery to discuss his or her fears or concerns. Losing a part of your body and learning to wear a prosthesis — an artificial limb — is a life-changing experience. There are amputee support groups that help people going through this experience

to share their emotions and learn from others. Having a positive attitude makes a tremendous difference.

THE REMAINING LEG

If you have had an amputation of one foot or leg, you are at higher risk of losing the other foot or leg. The odds are against you: 38% of people with diabetes who lose a leg will lose the other leg within three years, and 50% of people with diabetes who lose a leg will not survive five years. These statistics are telling. The risks of losing a leg are higher than all forms of cancer COMBINED, excluding lung and pancreatic cancers.

You and your caregivers need to be trained to be extra vigilant in detecting problems early and taking appropriate action. Working together, you will determine how to best:

- Relieve pressure on your foot

- Correct your leg position for poor blood supply

- Treat infection

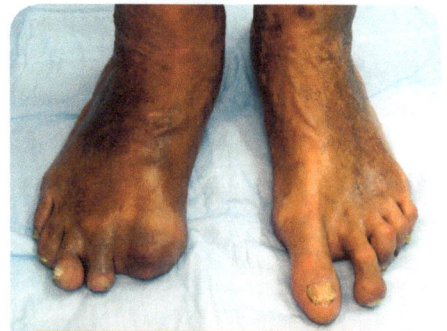

Digital Amputation

- Control blood sugars, blood lipids, blood pressure

- Quit smoking

- Practice preventive foot care behaviors

- Clean and dress foot wounds

- Secure ongoing professional foot care for treatment of corns, calluses and nails

- Prevent recurrence of foot ulcers

LIVING WITH AN AMPUTATION

Having an amputation changes your life. You may experience a sense of loss of personal liberty. You will have to expend 30 percent more energy walking and moving if you have a below-the-knee amputation and 60 percent more if you have an above-the-knee amputation.

Follow-up care

Taking care of your wound after your surgery is especially important to be sure the site heals without breakdown or infection. After the incision from the amputation site is healed, there can be swelling that can go on for six to eight weeks. To address the issue of edema (swelling) and to prepare the stump for a temporary prosthetic limb, you will likely have to wear a special elastic

FACTS

EVERY 30 MINUTES A LIMB IS LOST DUE TO A LANDMINE. EVERY 30 SECONDS, A LIMB IS LOST DUE TO DIABETES.

dressing called a "shrinker." When the swelling is reduced to a satisfactory level, you will be fitted with a temporary prosthetic limb. You will need to work with physical therapists in rehabilitation to learn how to balance and walk with only one leg or to push yourself in a wheelchair.

Financial Cost

The costs of amputation vary depending of the individual situation. So the numbers you see here may be higher or lower than the actual costs the day you read this book. A foot amputation can cost close to $30,000; a leg amputation can cost $60,000 or more, depending upon complications and other health care issues. The costs increase with the severity of the amputation, the length of hospitalization, and the need for rehabilitation, home care and social services. After hospitalization, its estimated three-year cost for home care and social services ranges from $30,000 to $60,000.

There are also indirect costs due to loss of productivity. Society as a whole pays in the form of higher insurance premiums or raised taxes to fund government programs that treat diabetes and its complications.

Accommodations

Life changes after you have an amputation. The life as you lived it before your amputation is no longer. You now have a "new normal." Adjustments will need to be made in your daily routine.

This is not an easy road, but you are not alone. You should get the help you need to keep a positive attitude so that you can accept the situation, work through it, and conscientiously follow your treatment plan.

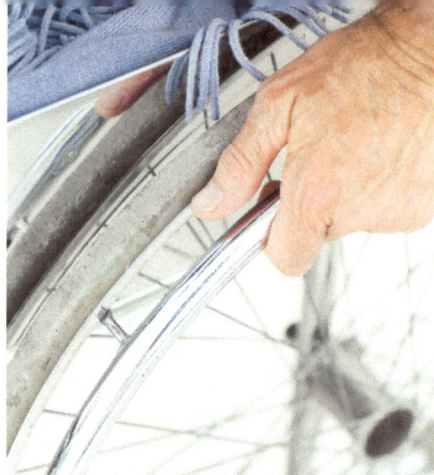

There are many accommodations for people with disabilities to help them continue to do gardening, cooking, traveling, etc. For transportation, there are vans outfitted with a motorized hoist to travel with a wheelchair or motorized scooter. There is handicapped parking and preferential seating at sporting and cultural events. You will have to learn to be patient and accept that, with a wheelchair or other accommodation, what you want to do will likely take a little extra time.

STATISTICS

The relative 5-year mortality rate after limb amputation is at least 50%. When compared with cancer — it is second only to lung cancer (86%). (Colorectal cancer 39%, Breast cancer 23%, Hodgkin's disease 18%, Prostate cancer 8%)

After a major amputation, 38% of people with diabetes will have their other limb amputated within 3 years.

Diabetes is attributed to about 80% of the 120,000 non-traumatic amputations performed yearly in the United States.

CHAPTER 18

PODIATRIC
MEDICINE

Podiatric Medicine is devoted to the study, diagnosis, and treatment of disorders of the foot, ankle, and lower leg. A Doctor of Podiatric Medicine (DPM) is a specialist qualified by education and training to diagnose and treat issues related to these areas.

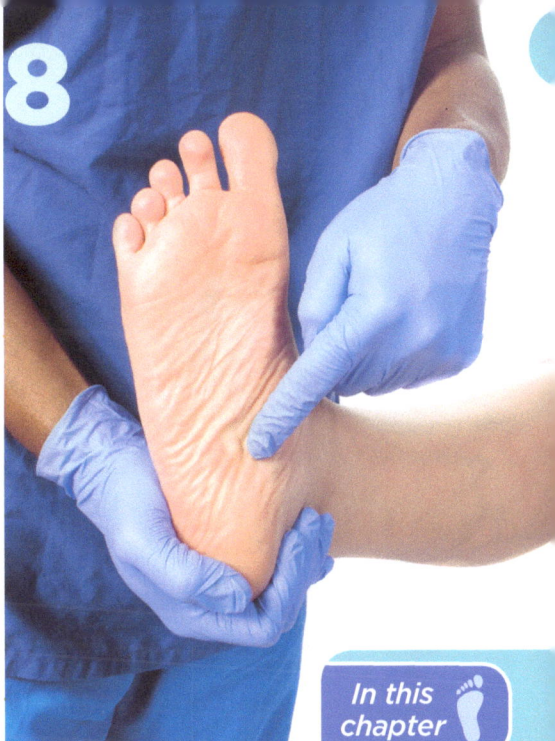

In this chapter

FOOT CARE
SPECIALIST

A
PODIATRIST'S
WORK

YOUR FOOT CARE SPECIALIST

The best thing about podiatric medicine is having the knowledge, education, training, skills and the proper tools to treat a wide variety of foot problems. A podiatrist is the best qualified health care professional to help you with special foot care issues and needs, especially if you are "at risk" for foot problems, and if you have poor circulation or peripheral arterial disease (PAD) and diabetes.

One of the most important services your podiatrist can offer is to educate you about how diabetes affects your feet. He or she can show you how a prevention plan can help maintain your foot health and prevent the terrible complications that diabetes can cause. This will give you a better quality of life and help control your health care costs.

FOOT CARE PROFESSIONAL

Foot care should be performed by a professional, licensed, qualified physician. Podiatric medicine started as podiatry and before that as chiropody. Chiropodists cut nails, trimmed corns and calluses and applied taping and padding for sore feet. With more advanced education, research and clinical training, podiatrists today are accepted members of the multidisciplinary team, which cares for the foot problems of people with diabetes. Today, there are eight schools of Podiatric Medicine in the United States, 213 residency-training programs approved by the Council on Podiatric Medical Education, and 14,000 podiatric physicians and surgeons. Today's graduating podiatrists may participate in 3-year residency programs and post-graduate fellowships in diabetes, limb salvage, sports medicine, arthritis and surgery. The 21st century podiatrist is the best trained and most well-prepared physician to handle any foot problem.

The education for doctors of podiatric medicine (DPM) is similar to other doctors. Students seeking to go into podiatric medical schools take the Medical College Admission Test (MCAT) required for entrance to all medical schools in the United States. In the first two years of their education, podiatric students study the same basic courses as all medical students. At the end of the first two years, podiatrists focus on intensive study of the lower extremities. These courses include medicine, surgery and biomechanics, the science that explains how foot structure affects foot function. With that education and post-graduate training, podiatrists learn to care for a wide variety of foot problems, including medical issues related to the skin, soft tissue, nails, gait and ambulation, and to deep structure of the foot, including the bones, deep soft tissue structures, and other metabolic and systemic foot conditions.

A PODIATRIST'S WORK

Podiatrists have a working knowledge of the nerves, circulation, and musculoskeletal systems of the foot and lower leg. They understand how the foot functions physically, physiologically, and biomechanically. They treat more than 300 possible diagnosable foot problems, including:

- Ankle and foot bone fractures, sprains, and strains, and foot injuries

- Arthritis and joint diseases

- Benign and malignant tumors

- Bone spurs, hammer toes, mallet toes, claw toes, and bunion deformities

- Corns and calluses

- Warts or plugged-up sweat gland ducts

- Diseased or ingrown toenails

- Foot complaints associated with diabetes, gout, ulcers, and peripheral arterial disease (PAD)

- Heel spurs/heel pain and arch problems

- Flat feet

- Nerve pain

- Problems of gait and ambulation

- Bacterial or fungal skin infections

- Limb length inequalities

These conditions may result from birth defects, heredity, trauma, improper shoes, abnormal gait, muscle and joint imbalances, or, as is the focus of this book, from diabetes.

PODIATRISTS HAVE A WORKING KNOWLEDGE IN ALL OF THE SYSTEMS OF THE FOOT AND LOWER LEG.

CHAPTER 19

YOUR MEDICAL TEAM

A multidisciplinary medical team is comprised of healthcare professionals from diverse disciplines whose goal of providing optimal patient care is achieved through coordination and communication with one another.

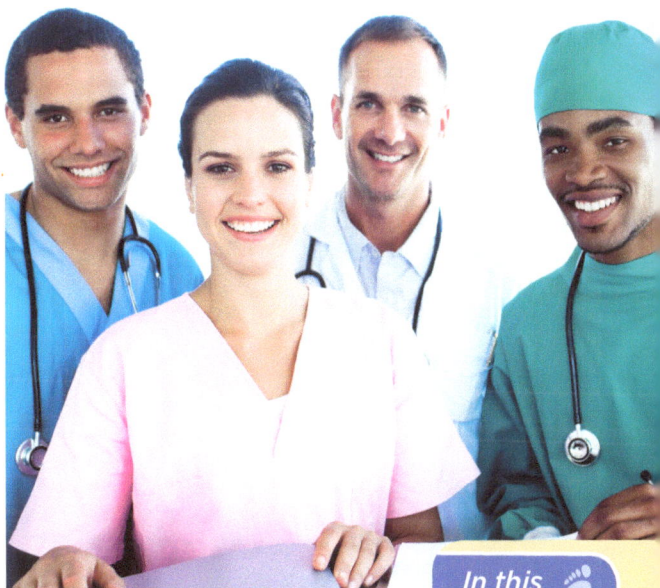

Your podiatrist will work with all of the other health care and medical professionals who will make up your health care team. Be sure that all those who are taking care of you are working together in coordinating your care. The following list can help you determine where to go for the kind of help you need and to understand the area of specialty of each member of the team.

- **Cardiologist:** A physician who specializes in diseases of the heart and blood vessels. For people with diabetes, a cardiologist may address problems related to circulation and blood pressure.

- **Certified Foot Care Nurse:** A member of the The Wound, Ostomy and Continence Nursing Certification Board who specializes in diabetic foot care.

- **Diabetes Educator:** (CDE-certified diabetes educator) A CDE is a health care professional who teaches people with diabetes how to manage their condition by learning the tools and skills necessary to control their blood sugar and avoid the long-term complications due to hyperglycemia or high blood sugars. Typically, the CDE is also a nurse, dietitian, pharmacist, or social worker who has further specialized in diabetes education and care management.

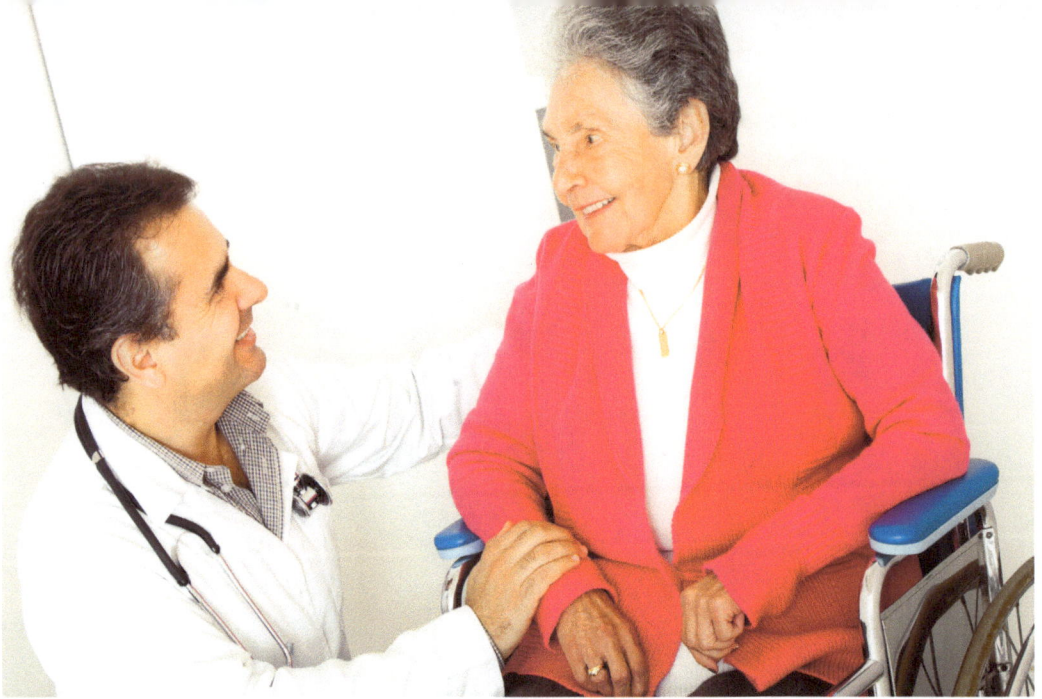

- **Nurse** (RN-registered nurse): A health care professional who has completed at least a two-or-four-year degree program in nursing, and who provides direct patient care for acutely or chronically ill patients. RNs may further specialize in a particular area.

- **Dietitian** (RD is a registered dietitian): Also called a nutritionist, this professional translates the science of nutrition into practical information about food. They work with people to promote nutritional well being, prevent food-related problems and treat disease. A dietitian who specializes in diabetes can provide you with a meal plan that is essential to managing your blood glucose. The meal plan can also address the vitamins and minerals you require to stay healthy.

- **Endocrinologist:** A physician who specializes in diseases of the internal glands of the body, an in treating diabetes. This specialist can help you to regulate your blood sugars with diet, exercise, and medications.

- **Infectious disease specialist:** A physician who specializes in the treatment of infections. This doctor can recommend antibiotics and monitor your organ functions while treating your infection.

- **Occupational Therapist (OT):** Occupational therapists help people overcome physical, psychological or social problems arising from illness or disability, by concentrating on what they are able to achieve, rather than on their disabilities This therapist can help you find devices, such as sock pullers and long-handed shoehorns, to accommodate your special needs.

- **Orthopedic Surgeon:** A physician who specialize in bone surgery; some orthopedic surgeons specialize in surgery of the foot and ankle.

- **Pharmacist (RPH):** A professional trained to prepare and distribute medicines and to give information about them. Pharmacists are familiar with medication ingredients, interactions, cautions, and hints.

- **Physical Therapist (PT)**: Physical therapists help people suffering from injury or disease to restore function, improve mobility, relieve pain, and prevent or limit permanent physical disabilities. PTs may use massage to improve muscle condition; apply ice to reduce swelling or heat to relieve pain; and use therapeutic equipment, such as whirlpool baths, ultrasonic machines, and ultraviolet and infrared lamps. They teach people how to exercise with pulleys and weights, stationary bicycles, and parallel bars. They also teach patients and their families how to use and care for wheelchairs, braces, canes and crutches, and artificial limbs. A PT might help people with diabetes who have trouble walking. If your require a cane, a PT can show you how to walk with it, and help to determine its proper length.

- **Physician Assistant:** A physician assistant helps prevent, maintain, and treat illnesses and injuries by providing health care services under the direction of a supervising physician. Similar to a physician, they can conduct physical exams, diagnose and treat illnesses, order and interpret tests, counsel on preventive health care, assist in surgery, and write prescriptions.

- **Pedorthist:** This professional evaluates people for fittings of custom-made shoes and insoles.

- **Primary Care Provider (PCP):** The physician responsible for the total health care of an individual and the family. This physician is usually a "general practice," "family practice" or an "internal medicine" physician.

BE SURE THAT ALL THOSE WHO ARE TAKING CARE OF YOU ARE WORKING TOGETHER IN COORDINATING YOUR CARE.

- **Prosthetist:** Prosthetists design and fit artificial replacements, called "prostheses." for upper and lower limbs. Orthotists make braces, splints and special footwear to help people with movement difficulties and to relieve discomfort.

- **Psychologist:** A professional specializing in diagnosing and treating diseases of the brain, emotional disturbance, and behavior problems through talk therapy.

- **Radiologist:** A physician who specializes in interpreting images including X-rays, computed tomography (CT) scans, ultrasound, and magnetic resonance imaging (MRI) and bone scans.

- **Vascular surgeon:** A physician who specializes in diseases of the chest, including lungs, heart, blood vessels and chest wall, that requires surgical operation for diagnosis and/or treatment. Some vascular surgeons further specialize in surgery on the blood vessels of the leg and foot.

RESOURCES

DIABETES AND THE FOOT

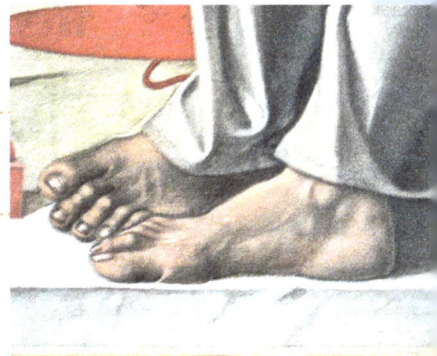

American Academy of Orthopaedic Surgeons
www.aaos.org

American Academy of Podiatric Sports Medicine
Specialists devoted to evaluating and managing lower extremity sports injuries
www.aapsm.org

American Association of Diabetes Educators
www.diabeteseducator.org

American Board of Podiatric Surgery
www.abps.org

American College of Foot and Ankle Surgeons
Surgically trained specialists devoted to evaluating and managing lower extremity injuries
www.acfas.org

American College of Sports Medicine
A diverse group of medical professionals with an interest in sports medicine
www.acsm.org

American Diabetes Association
www.diabetes.org

American Orthopaedic Foot and Ankle Society
www.aofas.org

The American Podiatric Medical Association
Foot and ankle specialists trained to evaluate and treat a wide array of lower extremity conditions.
www.apma.org

The American Professional Wound Care Association
www.apwca.com

American Running and Fitness Association
People with a common interest in improving running and fitness.
www.americanrunning.org

Center for Disease Control/Diabetes Control Division
www.cdc.gov/diabetes/pubs/tcyd/foot.htm

Clinical Trials/National Institutes of Health
Listing of clinical trials related to diabetes and foot care.
www.clinicaltrials.gov/ct2/results?term=diabetic+foot

The Diabetes Exercise and Sports Association and Insuline Independence
www.insulinindependence.org

d-Life
Dictionary of terms related to diabetes for the lay person.
A resource for active people with diabetes.
E-Newsletter on topics of health and diabetes.
www.dlife.com

Diabetes Health Professional
General information about diabetes sponsored by Life-Med Media.
www.diabeteshealth.com

The Diabetes Mall, San Diego
www.diabetesnet.com/diabetes

The International Working Group for the Diabetic Foot
Classification system for diabetic foot infection.
www.idf.org

Lower Extremity Amputation Prevention Program (LEAP)
www.bphc.hrsa.dhhs.gov/leap

Medicare/United States Department of Health and Human Services
Search for information on coverage for diabetic foot care.
www.medicare.gov

National Diabetes Education Program
www.ndep.nih.gov

National Institute of Diabetes and Digestive and Kidney Diseases.
National Diabetes Information Clearinghouse
www.niddk.nih.gov

National Odd Shoe Exchange (Phoenix)
www.oddshoe.org

National Patient Advocate Foundation
A national network to help people with access and advocacy for health care.
www.npaf.org/

Neuropathy Association
www.neuropathy.org

P.A.D. Coalition (Peripheral Arterial Disease)
www.padcoalition.org/wp

Pedorthic Footcare Association
www.pedorthics.org/

The Podiatry Channel
Part of Health Communities.com
www.podiatrychannel.com

Prevention First
www.prevention.com

Quack Watch
A guide to health fraud, quackery and making intelligent healthcare decisions.
www.quackwatch.org

Web MD
www.webmd.com

Emedicine health
(Part of Web MD)
www.emedicinehealth.com

LIMB SALVAGE CENTERS
Hospital-based centers for wound care, hyperbaric oxygen therapy and limb salvage

Alabama Limb Salvage Center
Shelby Baptist Medical Center
Alabaster, AL
www.alabamalimbsalvagecenter.com/

Amputation Prevention Center
Valley Presbyterian Hospital
Van Nuys, CA
www.valleypres.org/Amputation_
Prevention_Center

**Center for Wound Healing and
Hyperbaric Medicine**
Georgetown University Hospital
Washington, D.C.
www.georgetownuniversityhospital.
org/body_dept_home.cfm?id=513

Cleveland Clinic Limb Salvage Service
Cleveland, OH
www.clevelandclinic.org/services/
limb-salvage

**Comprehensive Wound & Disease
Management Center**
St. James Hospital
Chicago Heights, IL
www.stjameshospital.org/services/
wound_diseasemanagement.asp

International Center for Limb Salvage
Geneva, Switzerland
www.gfmer.ch/ICLS/Homepage.htm

Limb Salvage and Wound Care Center
Dallas Medical Center
Dallas, TX
www.cylex-usa.com/company/the
wound-andlimb-salvage-center-at-
dallas-medical-center17587719.html

Limb Salvage Center Washington
Hospital Center
Washington, D.C.
www.whcenter.org/

**New York Hyperbaric and Wound
Healing Center / St. Joseph Hospital**
New Island Hospital
Bethpage, NY
www.newislandhospital.org/

Southern Arizona Limb Salvage
Alliance University Medical Center
Tucson, AZ
http://surgery.arizona.edu/unit/center/
southern-arizona-limb-salvage-
alliance-salsa

Temple Limb Salvage Center
Temple University Hospital
Philadelphia, PA
http://tuh.templehealth.org/content/
limb_salvage.htm

**The American Diabetic Limb
Salvage Institute**
Dubai Healthcare City
Dubai, UAE
www.thelimbsalvageinstitute.com/

**The Joslin-Beth Israel Deaconess
Foot Center**
Beth Israel Deaconess Medical Center
Joslin Diabetes Center
Boston, MA
www.bidmc.org/Centersand
Departments/Departments/Surgery/
Podiatry.aspx

UNC Wound Health Center
University of North Carolina
Health Care
Chapel Hill, NC
www.unchealthcare.org/site/
woundmanagement

Wound Care Center/Center for Limb Salvage

Roper St. Francis Heart & Vascular Center
Charleston, SC
www.ropersaintfrancis.com

Wound Healing Center

Henry Piedmont Hospital
Stockbridge, GA
http://piedmonthenry.org/services/wound

The International Working Group for the Diabetic Foot on classification system for diabetic foot infections

Executive Office

Avenue Emile de Mot, 19
B-1000 Brussels, Belguim
Telephone: +32-2-5385511
E-mail: info@idf.org
Web site: www.idf.org

Internet Sites for More Information on Prevention

www.amputationprevention.com

www.apma.org

www.diabetes.org

www.diabetesnet.com/diabetes

www.emedicinehealth.com

www.padcoalition.org/wp/

www.podiatrychannel.com

www.prevention.com

www.webmd.com

Herbal and Dietary Supplements

www.itmonline.org/arts/diabherb.htm

www.diabetesmellitus-information.com/diabetes_herbs.htm

www.heartspring.net/diabetes_cinnamon.html

www.nutritionexpress.com

www.gymnema.net/

www.endocrinologist.com/herbs.html

Food and Nutrition

www.healingwithnutrition.com/ddisease/diabetes/diabetes.html

Kidney Disease

Diabetes is the leading cause of new cases of end-stage renal disease, accounting for about 40 percent of new cases.

www.vapodiatry.com/Medical_info.html

Blindness

Diabetes is the leading cause of new cases of blindness in adults 20 to 74 years of age. Each year 12,000 to 24,000 people lose their sight because of diabetes.

www.vapodiatry.com/Medical_info.html

HEALTH RESOURCES

Administration on Aging (AOA)
U.S. Department of Health and Human Services. Site with geriatric resources for professionals, patients and caregivers. Translations in German, Spanish, French, Italian, Korean, Japanese, Chinese and Portuguese.

Advanced Approaches to Chronic Pain Management
Medscape. Site dedicated to managing intractable pain.

Alternative Medicine Foundation
The Alternative Medicine Foundation is no longer operating as a nonprofit organization. The information resources compiled from 1998 to August 2010 have been retained on this web site as an archival resource but will not be further updated as of September 15, 2010.

Authentic Happiness
University of Pennsylvania- Philadelphia, Pennsylvania. A site focused on the study of positive motions, strength-based character and healthy institutions.

BenefitsCheckUp
The National Council on Aging. Resources for seniors to find benefit programs.

Center for Food Safety and Applied Nutrition
U.S. Food and Drug Administration (FDA). Nutrition resource.

Child Nutrition. Medline Plus
National Library of Medicine (NLM.) Resource for child nutrition.

CKD Insights
Site for searching for educational materials on renal disease, peritoneal dialysis, drug interactions and dialysis of drugs.

Clinical Trials.gov (NIH)
National Institute of Health (NIH).

Coalition on Donation-Donate Life
A non-proift alliance of organizations promoting organ, eye and tissue donation.

Consumer Health Library
Healthology is the leading producer and distributor of physician-generated health and medical information on the Internet. With the largest and most distinguished library of original, streaming health programs and physician-authored articles.

Cultural Competence Resources for Health Care Providers
Health Resources and Services Administration. U.S. Department of Health and Human Services.

Drugs, Supplements and Herbal Information
Medline Plus. National Library of Medicine (NLM). Comprehensive index site.

Eldercare Locator
U.S. Department of Health and Human Services. Extensive Information on senior services.

The Eldercare Team
Site for eldercare caregivers on questions and answers resources and support.

Factline
National Library of Medicine (NLM) Meharry Medical College. Health disparities faced by women minority groups and the elderly.

Food and Nutrition Information Center (FNIC)
Extensive nutritional resources.

Foot and Ankle Library
Formerly known as The Podiatric Medicine & Surgery Network, this web page contains links to all of the podiatry-related websites that we think you would be interested in seeing.

Free Medical Journals
Access to online free and full text journals.

Geriatric Care Medscape
Site for geriatric resources.

Geriatrics and Aging
Educational site that addresses health concerns of older adults.

Gilbert Guide
Resource of information on senior care facilities and resources.

Health Assistance Partnership
Site to help Medicare beneficiaries with health care.

Helping with Prescription Drug Costs
Social Security Online. Resource for Medicare beneficiaries who may qualify for prescription assistance if they have limited income and resources.

Hypertension Online
Baylor College of Medicine-Houston, Texas. Educational site for hypertension/blood pressure.

Infection Control in Healthcare Settings
Centers for Disease Control and Prevention (CDC). Resource for Healthcare-Associated Infections, Protecting Patients, Protecting Healthcare Workers, and Infection Control Guidelines.

Kid's Nutrition
Baylor College of Medicine- Houston, Texas. Resource for children's nutrition.

Lowering Your Blood Pressure with DASH (Dietary Approaches to Stop Hypertension)
National Heart Lung and Blood Institute. Dietary guidelines for blood pressure reduction.

MD Anderson Hospital
Complementary/Integrative Medicine Education Resource.

MDChoice.com
Medical Information Finder.

Medicare
U.S. Department of Health and Human Services. Comprehensive site for Medicare resources.

Medicare Central Families USA
Consumer health information on Medicare.

Medicare en Espanol
Partnership for Prescription Assistance

Medicare Prescription Drug Plan Medline Plus
National Library of Medicine (NLM). Resources on Medicare prescription drug coverage.

Medicare Rights Center
Information on Medicare.

Medicare Social Security Online
Resources on Medicare.

MedlinePlus/National Library of Medicine
Search engine for health topics, conditions and diseases.

My Pyramid
U.S. Department of Agriculture (USDA). Site with resources to help improve nutrition.

National Anemia Action Council
Resource for anemia patients and professionals.

National Center for Complementary and Alternative Medicine
National Institutes of Health (NIH). Site that reviews complementary and alternative medicine research, clinical trials and health information.

National Diabetes Education Program
NDEP is a partnership of the National Institutes of Health, the Centers for Disease Control and Prevention, and more than 200 public and private organizations.

National Institute of Neurological Disorders and Stroke (NINDS)
Reference page with extensive links on many diseases including Alzheimer's Disease.

National Patient Advocate Foundation
Site for National Network for Healthcare Access and patient advocacy information.

Needy Meds
Resource for prescription medicine assistance.

The New England Journal of Medicine
Source for clinical materials grouped by publisher.

The New York State Smoker's Quitsite
Smoking cessation.

NIH
U.S. Department of Health and Human Services/National Institutes of Health (NIH).

Nutrition.gov
U.S. Department of Agriculture (USDA). Site for online access on information on nutrition.

Nutrition and Fitness, Kids Health, Nemours Foundation
Resource for parents on kids' nutrition and fitness.

Office of Minority Health (CDC)
Centers for Disease Control ad Prevention (CDC). Reference site.

The Office of Minority Health (HHS)
The Department of Health and Human Services. Site focused on improving and protecting the health of racial and ethnic minority populations.

Overweight and Obesity
Centers for Disease Control and Prevention (CDC). Obesity review.

QuitNet
Boston University Smoking cessation site.

RxAssist
Resource of patient assistance programs on free and low-cost medications.

RxHope
Online patient assistance portal to locate patient pharmaceutical assistance programs.

RxMed
Reference site for Pharmaceutical Information and Herbal & Dietary Supplements.

Senior Citizens' Resources
Extensive resources for seniors.

Smokefree.gov
Resource for smoking cessation.

Smoking Cessation
Medline plus National Library of Medicine (NLM).

State Pharmaceutical Assistance Programs
Medicare. Resource by state for prescription assistance resources.

The Stretching Handbook
Site with Stretching Exercises.

United Network for Organ Sharing (UNOS)
A private, non-profit organization that manages the nation's organ transplant system under contract with the federal government.

Weight Control Medline Plus National Library of Medicine (NLM)
Resources for weight management.

Wolters Kluwer - Skin Care
Advances in Skin & Wound Care focuses on presenting new clinical research developments and providing practical information to help skin and wound care professionals better manage their clinical practice and make informed patient care decisions.

www.pubmed.com
Medical literature search site

effective 6/16/12

A

This book has been a labor of love for me, and I hope you the reader have enjoyed it and have learned from it. If you have only found one or two "nuggets" of information that will make the quality of your life better, and prevent the terrible complications that diabetes can bring to your feet, then my mission has been accomplished.

Prevention is beginning to show the promise of better foot health for those who practice it. The number of lower extremity amputations among people with diabetes has plummeted in recent years. According to a report in February, 2012, by the US Centers for Disease Control and Prevention, the rate of non-traumatic foot and leg amputations among adults with diagnosed diabetes fell by 65% between 1996 and 2008. Still the news isn't all good. Despite the earlier diagnosis of foot and leg problems and better care, diabetes-related amputation is still about eight times higher than the rate among non-diabetic people.

While medical science continues to fit the pieces of the puzzle of diabetes together and searches for a cure, people with diabetes continue to suffer the complications of the disease to their legs and feet.

Please remember that you need not suffer the complications of diabetes when it comes to your feet if you choose to learn about your foot health and practice preventive foot health behaviors.

Dr. Mark Hinkes, DPM

www.ingramcontent.com/pod-product-compliance
Lightning Source LLC
Chambersburg PA
CBHW060800270326
41926CB00002B/42